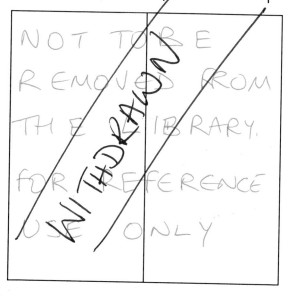

D1340005

For Churchill Livingstone:

Publisher: Laurence Hunter
Project Editor: Janice Urquhart
Copy Editor: Colin Macnee
Project Controller: Nancy Arnott
Design Direction: Erik Bigland

A Manual of English
for the Overseas Doctor

Joy Parkinson BA

Former Head of the Department of English,
Southwark College, London

FIFTH EDITION

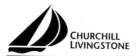

EDINBURGH LONDON NEW YORK PHILADELPHIA SAN FRANCISCO SYDNEY
TORONTO 1999

CHURCHILL LIVINGSTONE
An imprint of Harcourt Brace and Company Limited

© Longman Group 1991
© Harcourt Brace and Company Limited 1999

⟁ is a registered trade mark of Harcourt Brace and Company Limited

The right of Joy Parkinson to be identified as author of this work has been asserted by her in accordance with the Copyright, Designs and Patents Act 1988.

First edition 1969
Second edition 1976
Third edition 1985
Fourth edition 1991
Fifth edition 1999

ISBN 0 443 06136 X

British Library of Cataloguing in Publication Data
A catalogue record for this book is available from the British Library.

Library of Congress Cataloging in Publication Data
A catalog record for this book is available from the Library of Congress.

Medical knowledge is constantly changing. As new information becomes available, changes in treatment, procedures, equipment and the use of drugs become necessary. The author and the publishers have, as far as it is possible, taken care to ensure that the information given in this text is accurate and up to date. However, readers are strongly advised to confirm that the information, especially with regard to drug usage, complies with current legislation and standards of practice.

The
publisher's
policy is to use
**paper manufactured
from sustainable forests**

Produced by Addison Wesley Longman China Limited, Hong Kong
GCC/01

Preface

The first edition of this book was published in 1969 to meet the needs of a continuing flow of overseas doctors coming to the UK for specialist training. At that time most were from countries like India, Pakistan, Egypt and Iraq where medical education was in English. However, the language spoken by patients in hospitals in the UK is vastly different from that used overseas. Hence a large part of the book is concerned with the vocabulary and language used in the doctor–patient relationship.

In the thirty years since the publication of the first edition and the preparation of the fifth much has changed. The National Health Service has been reorganised several times, some institutions have disappeared, others merged and new ones appeared, the number of medical abbreviations has multiplied enormously and drug use for recreational purposes has spread to unthinkable limits. Perhaps, most important of all, attitudes have changed: we have undergone a social revolution and this is reflected in the use of language.

What has not changed is the flow of doctors from all over the world to the UK for observation of new techniques, for specialist training and for preparation for work in our hospitals. Political upheavals in various parts of the world have forced many doctors to seek refuge and work here. Faced with a new language and a new culture, they need all the support possible in re-establishing themselves.

I have had the privilege of teaching medical English to hundreds of doctors from all parts of the globe. From them I have learned so much. Their appreciation of the *Manual* and their suggestions for improvements have been a source of pleasure and encouragement to me. There are now Chinese, Japanese and Polish editions available.

I hope that this new edition, which has been completely revised with many new case histories, will be of great help to those doctors arriving in the new millennium.

Joy Parkinson   London 1998

Acknowledgements

As with the four previous editions of the *Manual*, many people have given me necessary specialist help.

Dr Peter Bourdillon kindly gave me advice on the structure of the National Health Service and hospital medical staffing. Neil Edgar, David Foster and Grainne Kelly of the Whittington Hospital helped me to up-date the chapter on the organisation of a hospital. Thanks are due to Philip Carter, Assistant Dean of Postgraduate Medicine (Overseas Doctors) of the North Thames Department of Postgraduate Medical Education for his patient help with all the changes in this field. Dr Fiona Godlee, Assistant Editor of the British Medical Journal, guided me through the enormous number of new medical abbreviations. I received help from the Institute for the Study of Drug Dependence and from Paddy Screech of the Hungerford Drug Project on the complexities of the language of drug culture. Thanks are also due for advice from Sam McCarter and Doug Young of Southwark College and Penny Layton of Relate.

Over the years I have received invaluable help from the staff of the Whittington Hospital — secretaries, librarians, nurses, doctors, all busy people but appreciating the fact that overseas doctors coming to this country need help.

I should like to thank particularly the following for advice, encouragement and permission to publish information and case histories: Dr Celia Bielawska, Dr Kenneth Earle, Dr Frederika Eben, Dr Portia Goldsmith, Mr Eric Heaton, Dr Norman Johnson, Dr Anna Karowska, Dr Gill Livingstone, Dr Clare McLure and Dr Peter Moult.

In addition thanks are due to Dr G. D. Perkin of the Charing Cross Hospital.

ACKNOWLEDGEMENTS

My special gratitude must, as in the previous four editions, go to Dr Eric Beck, Consultant Physician at the Whittington Hospital, who has been a great source of encouragement to me from the beginning. He was the first doctor to allow me to record case histories, he put me in touch with other doctors and most important he believed in what I was trying to do.

My thanks to Zena Austin for patiently typing the new material.

Contents

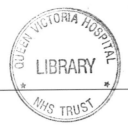

Note on weights and measures

Although the UK has officially adopted the metric system of weights and measures, many people still use the former system so it is important to understand both:

1 ounce (oz) = 28.35 grams
16 oz = 1 pound (lb) = 0.454 kilograms
14 lb = 1 stone (st) = 6.356 kilograms

1 inch (in) = 2.54 cm
12 in = 1 foot (ft) = 30.479 cm
3 feet = 1 yard (yd) = 0.9144 m

Temperature equivalents:
To convert degrees Fahrenheit (°F) to degrees Celsius or centigrade (°C) subtract 32 and multiply the remainder by 5/9.

98.6°F = 37°C

The structure of the National Health Service

On 6 November 1946 the National Health Service Act, after passing through Parliament, received the Royal Assent and was brought into operation on 5 July 1948. Since that date the people of the UK have been able to make use of one of the most elaborate, most comprehensive health services in the world. The NHS, a multi-billion pound enterprise, is the country's largest employer with about one million workers.

The money for the NHS comes mainly from general taxation but all employed people make some contribution to the cost of the service through their weekly National Insurance payments. Most medical treatment is free but charges are made for some items, including drugs, spectacles and dental care; these services are free for children, the elderly, the chronically sick and the unemployed. Free emergency medical treatment is given to any visitor from abroad who becomes ill whilst in this country but those who come to England specifically for treatment must pay for it.

An interesting aspect of the NHS is that the patient can choose between NHS or private treatment at any time; moreover, he can take one part with the service, the other privately. So, he may go to a NHS doctor but to a dentist privately. If a patient is dissatisfied with his NHS family doctor or dentist, he may change to another one. In fact, more than 90% of the population use the NHS in some form. Only about 10% of hospital care is provided from the private sector.

This freedom of choice applies to doctors and dentists too. They are able to choose whether they want to join the NHS or not, and if they wish they can have NHS and private patients. In fact, the majority work in the service.

RECENT CHANGES IN STRUCTURE

A number of major changes in the organisation of the NHS have taken place in recent years.

Government policy in the White Paper, 'Working for Patients', presented to Parliament in 1989, added the concept of an internal market within the NHS. Another White Paper, 'Caring for People: Community care in the next decade and beyond', published in 1989, proposed major changes in long-term hospital care.

In 1996 a White Paper, 'Developing a Primary Care Led NHS' stated that the objective was to ensure that health care decisions were taken as close to patients as possible, with a greater say for patients and their carers in those decisions.

THE PRESENT STRUCTURE

The Department of Health

The Secretary of State for Health is the head of the Department of Health (DoH). This is a political appointment. The staff of the Department of Health are civil servants. The Secretary of State is responsible to Parliament for the NHS, and officers of the DoH assist him in major policy decisions.

Function
The work of the DoH is to assist the Secretary of State in the following ways:
— to decide the kind, scale and balance of service to be provided in regions;
— to guide and support the Health Authorities and to allocate to them the necessary resources;
— to provide a specialist contribution on personnel, finance, property and building supply;
— to carry out some research and to prepare national statistics;
— to support the Secretary of State in his Parliamentary and public duties.

Health Authorities

On 1 April 1996 100 Health Authorities (HAs) were set up. These HAs are able to develop comprehensive strategies across all primary care, hospital and community services. One of their key responsibilities is to work in partnership with all General Practitioners (GPs) and other providers such as dentists, community pharmacists, nurses and optometrists to develop local strategies and to purchase high-quality services to meet the needs of local patients.

Family Health Services

The Family Health Services provide most of the day-to-day health care needed by the community, and for most people they are the regular point of contact with the NHS.

These services include those provided by GPs, dentists, pharmacists and optometrists, who are independent but work under contract to the NHS. Their role includes identifying and referring patients who need more specialised investigation or care. Making appropriate referrals is a major factor in the effective functioning of the secondary care (hospital) services.

General Practitioners

Under the NHS everyone should register with a local General Practitioner (GP), sometimes called a family doctor because it is usual for the doctor to see all members of the family.

GPs are heavily involved in commissioning health care for local people and ensuring that people have access to hospital care, community care, physiotherapy, management of drug addiction and other services.

Social services

Social services, often called community care, dealing with problems such as housing for people with physical disabilities and domestic help for the sick and elderly, are planned and controlled by local government authorities. The cost of the social services comes mainly from local government funds. Although financed separately, it is very important that health and social services should be planned jointly, especially for the old, those with learning disabilities, sensory disabilities and the mentally ill. Under the 1973 Act there is a statutory responsibility for all health authorities to plan with the corresponding local government authorities and this has been strengthened by recent legislation. This co-operation is vital to the success of the NHS.

Community Health Councils

The NHS Reorganisation Act 1973 set up Community Health Councils (CHCs). These CHCs represent the views of the people who use the NHS. There is one for each health district. Half of the CHC membership is appointed by local authorities, one third is nominated by voluntary organisations and the rest are appointed by the Secretary of State. There are usually from 18 to 24 members, who are unpaid but may claim expenses. They have direct access to the Minister on changes in the health services.

Function
A CHC's main task is to represent to its HA the interests of the public in the health service in its district. It has the power to seek information, to inspect hospitals, the right to consult senior officers of the HAs and to get information from them, and the duty to issue annual reports. It is also able to help patients with grievances.

Health Service Commissioner

Another feature of the NHS is the Health Service Commissioner (Ombudsman) who investigates certain complaints, including clinical competence, against NHS authorities The Health Service has formal procedures for complaints against doctors. The procedure has three stages: local resolution, the appointment of external assessors, the Ombudsman. These procedures are operated by the

General Managers of the Units in which they work. A person who wishes to complain can contact a Commissioner directly but he cannot investigate a complaint until the health authority concerned has investigated the matter. If after receiving a reply the person is still dissatisfied and the complaint is within his jurisdiction, as defined by Statute, the Commissioner may investigate it further.

The organisation of a hospital

The management of hospitals is organised by the Chief Executive of a Trust who is accountable to the Trust Board of the hospitals concerned. Moreover, management is increasingly being designed on the basis that decisions and control of resources are delegated to the lowest appropriate level within the organisation.

In many hospitals Clinical Directorates (or groups with the same function with different names) are the main unit of management which doctors will encounter. These Directorates are responsible for the care of a particular group of patients looked after by a specialty or a group of specialties. In other hospitals, this reorganisation has not gone so far and there is still a more centralised structure with assistants to the Chief Executive dealing with specific services, such as Inpatients or Outpatients.

In running the hospital, the Chief Executive will have the benefit of a team of Senior Managers with medical, nursing and other professional advice who will meet together to co-ordinate services.

THE STAFF OF A HOSPITAL

Medical staff

The range of medical posts in a hospital, from the most senior to the most junior are:
— *Career grades*
  — Consultant
  — Associate Specialist
  — Staff Grade

— *Trainee grades*
— Specialist Registrar
— Senior House Officer
— Pre-registration House Officer.

Consultant

Consultants are appointed having gained a Certificate of Completion of Specialist Training (CCST) and having been successful at an Advisory Appointments Committee. The Consultant, the most senior grade in medical posts, has the ultimate decision on patient care.

A consultancy is a permanent post but it can be full time or part time, allowing a doctor to spend some time in private practice.

Part-time appointments are calculated in terms of half-day sessions of $3\frac{1}{2}$ hours. Both full and part-time consultants may work on a sessional basis at more than one hospital.

In order to be a consultant the highest qualifications are required, including, for example, postgraduate diplomas such as FRCS for surgery, the MRCP for physicians and accreditation by the appropriate higher specialist training committee of one of the Royal Colleges. The male surgeons are addressed as Mr* X and the female surgeons as Miss or Mrs[†] Y; the other consultants as Doctor Z.

Associate Specialist

Doctors in this grade have considerable experience. They are nominally under the supervision of a consultant.

Staff Grade

Staff Grade posts were created in 1987 to find ways of providing essential support to consultants in the acute specialties without training doctors for non-existent posts. The Specialist Training Authority will not recognise time spent in a Staff Grade post as part of training. This makes the chance of obtaining a CCST and

---

*pronounced 'mister', but never written this way.
[†]Pronounced 'missis', but never written this way.

hence a consultancy small. The promotion that is open is to Associate Specialist.

Specialist Registrar

Specialist Registrars are the result of the Calman Report recommending structured training and a merging of the Registrar and Senior Registrar grades. Specialist Registrars are undertaking Higher Specialist Training. The duration of the training varies according to the specialty, e.g. 4 years for anaesthetics and 6 years for cardiology. As with the consultants, the Surgical Specialist Registrar would be addressed as Mr X, Miss or Mrs Y and the others as Dr Z.

A Surgical Specialist Registrar will do the routine surgery, for example, appendicectomy, hernia etc, without the supervision of a more senior surgeon but he will only perform major operations with a more senior surgeon present.

Senior House Officers

Senior House Officers (SHOs) are undertaking Basic Specialist Training. This lasts for 2–3 years until they are successful in obtaining a Specialist Registrar post. If unsuccessful, SHOs can apply for Staff Grade posts. Appointments may be for periods of 6 months upwards and such posts are frequently part of a rotating training scheme. SHOs look after the routine medical care of the patient.

Pre-registration House Officers

Since 1953 it has been compulsory for newly qualified doctors to serve one year as a pre-registration house officer before being admitted to the Register. Pre-registration posts exist in the majority of general hospitals. These doctors are considered in law to be doctors only for the purpose of a specific post. They have clinical responsibility but under supervision.

Nursing staff

Approximately 10% of nursing staff in NHS hospitals are men. The percentage is much higher in mental hospitals. It is difficult to recognise the different grades of the nursing staff of a hospital since every hospital is free to choose its own uniform. In addition, many senior nursing staff no longer wear uniform. However, although the dress worn by nursing staff differs from hospital to hospital, the grades are similar but a wide range of titles are now being used to describe similar jobs. They are as follows.

Chief Nurse

This post carries the overall responsibility for nursing policy and practice within hospitals. Commonly the post may also involve a general management or quality assurance function. This is the most senior nurse in the hospital. The Chief Nurse has a seat on the Executive Board. Other titles that are used to describe this post are Nurse Director, Executive Nurse and sometimes Director of Nursing.

Senior Nurse

There may be several Senior Nurses within a hospital who have responsibility for the management of a group of wards or department within a specific clinical service such as those for elderly people, the mentally ill or patients needing intensive care. The Senior Nurses are usually responsible to General Managers for the day-to-day running of services and to the Chief Nurse for professional issues affecting nursing care. The Senior Nurses themselves may be general managers and have titles reflecting this, such as Service Manager or Assistant General Manager.

Clinical Nurse Specialists

These nurses are highly qualified and experienced. They specialise in an aspect of nursing in parallel to medical staff, often taking their own groups of patients through a range of treatments without reference to a doctor (they are highly autonomous practitioners). They may also be known as nurse practitioners. This is the commonest title for these nurses in Accident and Emergency Departments where they have the authority to assess, treat and discharge patients with minor injuries.

Ward Sister or Charge Nurse

The Ward Sister (female) or Charge Nurse (male) has responsibility for running and organising a ward or department. In formal situations the titles Sister or Charge Nurse (or Mr X) may be used, but otherwise first names are considered appropriate. It is increasingly common that the title given to these posts is Ward Manager to indicate that the job includes managing all the services focused on the ward and its patients.

Staff Nurse

Staff Nurses are qualified nurses who are responsible to the Ward Sister or Charge Nurse. This is the first post newly qualified nurses will hold, but some Staff Nurses are highly experienced and often have specialist qualifications relevant to their ward area.

Enrolled Nurse

Enrolled Nurses are experienced and fully qualified nurses who often perform nursing care rather than taking responsibility for running the ward. They undertook a 2 year training which has now been discontinued.

Student Nurses

These are nurses in training with a university. They will be allocated to hospital settings to gain clinical experience.

Nursing qualifications

There are a number of nursing qualifications that are gained through university education. The pre-registration programme lasts three years and leads to registration through four branches: adult, child, mental health and learning difficulties. Each of these specialities results in registration as an RN (Registered Nurse).

Health Care Assistants

Health Care Assistants work with Registered Nurses and undertake basic patient care under the direction of qualified staff. It is increasingly common that Health Care Assistants collect evidence in recognition of their practical abilities and experience of looking after patients, which results in accreditation that may lead them to enter education to work towards nursing qualifications.

Paramedical staff

In addition to the medical and nursing staff of a hospital there are many other people who work in the allied professions, including the following.

Chiropodists
Treatment under the NHS is mainly for the elderly.

Dietitians
Most hospitals have one or more dietitians and facilities for the preparation of special diets. The dietitian will assist the medical staff by advising their patients on diets. In many hospitals the dietitian takes part in outpatient clinics to give advice to patients referred to her by consultants.

Pharmacists
All general hospitals will employ qualified pharmacists, and other specialist hospitals like psychiatric and mental handicap probably will too.

Physiotherapists
These people are trained to give treatment by massage, exercise, hydrotherapy and electrotherapy, to help restore specific bodily functions.

Remedial Gymnasts
These are involved in rehabilitation following operations and medical accidents, such as strokes. They help patients to over-come disabilities by the use of corrective exercises.

Occupational Therapists
These are found in many general hospitals and in all specialist

hospitals. They are extremely important in the work of rehabilitation by training patients in activities which help restore their mental and physical capability, and where this is not possible by assisting them overcome their handicaps by the provision of suitable aids.

Radiographers

Radiographers take X-rays and operate equipment in X-ray Departments for diagnostic purposes. Some radiographers who are specialists in radiotherapy treatment operate radiotherapy machines under the direction of radiotherapists.

Medical Laboratory Scientific Officers

These people work in departments responsible for the analysis of specimens.

Speech Therapists

Most hospitals employ at least one speech therapist who will see patients as part of their rehabilitation after strokes, etc.

Nearly all these members of hospital staff wear white coats but they frequently have labels to show their professional function. All paramedical staff except trainees must pass the appropriate professional examinations.

Social Workers

All social problems that have contributed to the patient's illness or that arise as a result of it are referred to the social workers.

The social workers spend much of their time in hospitals but since the 1974 Act they are part of the team of social workers employed by the Local Authority.

Administrative and Support Services staff

There are many other groups of staff employed within the hospital with whom the doctor will have less contact but who are equally essential to the functioning of the hospital. Amongst these are the domestic, catering and laundry staff, building and maintenance craftsmen and porters. These are often called the Support Services staff. Finally there are the administrative and clerical staff who work in a number of departments: medical records, salaries and wages, accounts, personnel and general administration.

Postgraduate medical training and registration

3

ADVISORY SERVICE

There has been a major restructuring of postgraduate medical training in order to conform to a European Union directive. Instead of Senior House Officer, Registrar and Senior Registrar posts, the Senior House Officer grade is constructed to be a specialist training post, and Registrar and Senior Registrar posts have been combined into Senior Registrar posts for specialist training. Formal curricula have been developed for all specialties although the length of training varies. **It is essential to seek advice at least 1 year before coming to the UK in order to obtain the necessary information and to allow sufficient time for subsequent action**.

The National Advice Centre for Postgraduate Medical Education (NACPME) was set up in 1989 to provide information to overseas-qualified doctors on postgraduate medical education and training in the UK. All British Council offices hold information on medical training in the UK and initial enquiries should be made to them. For those countries where there is no British Council office, doctors should write direct to:

National Advice Centre for Postgraduate Medical Education
Medlock Street
Manchester
M15 4AA
UK

MEDICAL REGISTRATION FOR OVERSEAS-QUALIFIED DOCTORS

An overseas-qualified doctor must apply to:

The General Medical Council
178 Great Portland Street
London
W1N 6JE
UK

for registration before engaging in any professional employment in the UK. Doctors wishing to work in the UK are advised to write to the General Medical Council (GMC) *at least 9 months* before they intend to leave their own countries. The GMC cannot help a doctor to find employment but by granting him registration it gives him the necessary legal status for carrying out his professional duties.

There are three types of registration: full, provisional and limited.

Full registration

A doctor who holds a qualification recognised by the GMC for the purpose of full registration may apply for this. Documentary evidence must be given that a doctor has obtained certain professional experience since qualifying.

Provisional registration

A doctor who holds a qualification recognised by the GMC for full registration but who has not had the necessary professional experience may apply for provisional registration. However, the number of posts in the UK suitable for doctors with provisional registration is so limited that doctors from overseas are urged not to come at an early stage in their training but to gain the necessary professional experience first.

European Economic Area (EEA)

A national of an EEA country who holds a recognised primary medical qualification granted in the EEA is eligible for full registration in the UK.

Limited registration

Limited registration may be granted to a doctor who holds a qualification, obtained overseas, which is accepted by the GMC for this purpose. Such registration may be held only in respect of supervised employment in approved hospitals or institutions and may be granted in relation to one particular employment or a specified range of employment. Limited registration is only granted for a period of 5 years.

PLAB test (Professional and Linguistic Assessments Board)

The majority of overseas doctors who wish to apply for limited registration for the first time will be required to pass the PLAB test. To be eligible to take the PLAB test, a doctor must have evidence of having satisfactorily completed an internship of 12 months' duration or an acceptable equivalent. Evidence is also required that a doctor has gained a satisfactory grade in the IELTS (p. 18).

Doctors who intend to seek sponsorship may be eligible for exemption from taking the PLAB test (see Sponsorship, page 21). The PLAB test is designed to assess overseas-qualified doctors' medical abilities and fluency in English before they are granted registration to work in the UK. The PLAB test comprises two parts: the medical and the Objective Structured Clinical Examination (OSCE) (see page 20).

Part 1

Medical component

This part consists of three medical, written papers:

1. the Multiple Choice Question examination (MCQ)
2. the Clinical Problem Solving examination

3. the Photographic Material examination.

1. *The Multiple Choice Question examination.* This is designed to test your factual medical knowledge and recall. There are 60 questions, each of five parts, to be done in the one and a half hours allotted. There are questions on medicine, surgery, obstetrics and gynaecology. The medicine questions include psychiatry, dermatology, community medicine, paediatrics, etc., so it is obviously necessary to revise these subject areas thoroughly.

2. *The Clinical Problem Solving examination.* This paper is designed to assess your ability to apply your professional knowledge to a variety of clinical situations, to interpret symptoms, signs and investigations and to give instructions for the care and management of patients. The examination consists of three problems, all of which must be attempted. Failure to do so means loss of marks and likely failure of the test. Questions cover the main branches of medicine: medicine, surgery, obstetrics and gynaecology and related disciplines.

3. *The Photographic Material examination.* This lasts 40 minutes and is designed to assess a candidate's knowledge by means of 20 photographs depicting various clinical conditions covering the three main branches of medical practice. They include clinical conditions, investigations including X-rays and ECGs, and clinical pathological material including blood films and operation and postmortem specimens.

From October 1997 it was possible for doctors to take the medical component in certain centres in India.

English language test (the IELTS)

The linguistic competence of prospective PLAB test candidates is now tested by the IELTS examination (The International English Language Testing System). This test is administered by the British Council at overseas centres throughout the world, including the UK.

The IELTS is recognized by higher education authorities

throughout the world as a measure of competence to study in the medium of English. It consists of four tests:

1. Listening
2. Reading
3. Writing
4. Speaking.

The first three tests are always taken in one day, with the speaking test on the same day or up to 2 days later.

1. *Listening*. This listening comprehension is designed to test your ability to understand spoken English. The tape lasts about 30 minutes and there are 40 questions to answer of varying difficulty. There are four sections to the test and you will hear several passages including male and female voices and a variety of accents. You will hear the passage ONCE ONLY as in most situations in real life. Your answers will be in a booklet and require notes, letters or numbers rather than continuous writing.

2. *Reading*. The reading test lasts 60 minutes and there are 40 questions to assess your ability to understand different types of texts. The question booklet has three reading passages, some of which contain graphs, tables or diagrams. There is a wide range of question types: some require complete sentences, others to fill gaps, answer multiple choice questions and so on. It is important that you control the time on each reading passage, and work fast in order to complete the questions.

3. *Writing*. The writing test lasts 60 minutes and there are two tasks to complete. In the first task you have to write a *description* of information usually given in a diagram or table. You have 20 minutes and have to write a minimum of 150 words. Your description has to be clear and logical.

   In the second task, you are presented with a point of view or argument or problem. Appropriate responses are short essays or general reports. You have 40 minutes and have to write a minimum of 250 words. It is very important to control your use of time. In this part, your answers must be written in complete sentences, not in note form. A booklet is provided in which to write your answers.

4. *Speaking*. The speaking test is an interview and lasts about 15 minutes. There are five parts and the first is to introduce yourself to the examiner. The second is on general topics such as your own experiences. In the third part you are given a card with some information and you are required to ask the examiner questions to elicit information or to solve a problem. In the fourth part you are asked about your future plans. The interview is then concluded. It is a test of your ability to communicate effectively with native speakers of English.

The IELTS is not an examination in which you pass or fail. You are given a band score which shows your ability in each of the four sections. The GMC requires a minimum overall band score of 7.0 in the IELTS test, with a minimum score of 6.0 in each of the four sections.

Part 2

The OSCE (Objective Structured Clinical Examination) forms the final stage of the assessment of doctors who have already achieved the required band score of IELTS and passed the medical component of PLAB. The OSCE is held three times a year in London and Edinburgh. The examination lasts 2 hours and tests communication skills, emergency life-saving techniques, medicine, surgery, obstetrics and gynaecology. Candidates go through a series of stations with a clearly stated time limit for each one. At each station the candidate is required to perform a particular task which could range from a partial physical examination of a patient to the discussion of the management of, for example, a patient with a myocardial infarction. The communication skills of the candidate are tested by such means as breaking bad news to a patient, advising on how to cope with a member of the family with Alzheimer's Disease, etc. Each task is marked objectively against a previously agreed marking chart.

Training to be a specialist

A doctor who wishes to train as a specialist in the UK requires experience and instruction in his chosen subject. The training programme should be carefully planned with the help of the appropriate Royal College and the Postgraduate Dean of any region.

Hospital employment

When a doctor has succeeded in passing the PLAB test or has obtained exemption from it, he may then apply for a post. Vacancies are advertised weekly in the Lancet and the British Medical Journal.

There is great competition for training posts in some specialties, especially general medicine, general surgery, paediatrics, and obstetrics and gynaecology. You should, therefore, not come to the UK unless you have sufficient money to live without working, as you cannot expect to find a post immediately.

SPONSORSHIP

Attention is drawn to the possibility of receiving a sponsorship. It is recommended that you try to gain a sponsorship before coming to the UK. It is necessary to apply to the Government of the country of which you are a national. Sponsorship may be obtained through a variety of channels, including the British Council, the Association of Commonwealth Universities and the World Health Organization. The Overseas Doctors Training Scheme (ODTS) is a sponsorship scheme for well-qualified doctors from overseas who have a good command of English. It is the home sponsors who make the application to the Royal College. Specific advice on sponsorship can be obtained from the General Medical Council (GMC).

POSTGRADUATE COURSES

Advice about training can be obtained by writing to the Advice Centre and to the Royal Colleges listed below. It should be noted that advanced courses are for those who have had experience for a long time in a specialist field.

MEDICAL DEFENCE INSURANCE

NHS hospitals have block indemnity insurance for their full-time doctors. However, overseas doctors are strongly recommended to take out supplementary indemnity insurance by writing to one of the following:

— Medical Defence Union, 3 Devonshire Place, London, W1N 2EA, UK.
— Medical Protection Society, 50 Hallam Street, London, W1N 6DE, UK.
— Medical and Dental Defence Union, 144 West George Street, Glasgow, G2 2HW, UK.

USEFUL BOOKS AND ADDRESSES

Books
— *A Book for IELTS* by Sam McCarter, Julie Easton and Judith Ash, published by IntelliGene.
— *A Book on Writing* by Sam McCarter, published by IntelliGene.
— *Cambridge Practice Tests for IELTS 1* by Vanessa Jakeman and Clare McDowell, published by Cambridge University Press.
— *Communication Skills for Medicine* by M. Lloyd and R. Bor, published by Churchill Livingstone.
— *IELTS Practice Now* by Carol Gibson, published by the Centre for Applied Linguistics in the University of South Australia, Adelaide.
— PLAB Medical MCQ practice papers.
— PLAB practice exams: Medical sections.
The above two books are available by post from PASTEST, Egerton Court, Parkgate Estate, Knutsford, Cheshire, WA16 8DX, UK.
— *The Duties of a Doctor*, published by the General Medical Council and available free of charge.

Courses

Courses preparing overseas doctors for PLAB are run by PASTEST in London. Courses preparing doctors for IELTS and Medical English are run by the Medical English Unit, at Southwark College, The Cut, Waterloo, London, SE1 8LE, UK. The Library at Southwark has a large reference section for the PLAB medical component.

Addresses

— British Council, 10 Spring Gardens, London, SW1A 2BN, UK.

— British Medical Association, Tavistock Square, London, WC1H 9JP, UK.

— Conference of Postgraduate Medical Deans of the UK, 33 Millman Street, London, WC1N 3EJ, UK.

— Conjoint Board (Ireland), The Secretary, Conjoint Board (Ireland), 123 St Stephen's Green, Dublin 2, Eire.

— Faculty of Public Health Medicine: The Secretary, Faculty of Public Health Medicine, 4 St Andrew's Place, London, NW1 4LB, UK.

— Faculty of Occupational Medicine: The Secretary, Faculty of Occupational Medicine, Royal College of Physicians of London, 6 St Andrew's Place, Regent's Park, London, NW1 4LB, UK.

— General Medical Council: The Registrar, General Medical Council, 178 Great Portland Street, London, W1N 6JE, UK Health Departments:

1. *England:* Department of Health, Richmond House, 79 Whitehall, London, SW1A 2NS, England.

2. *Wales:* The Health Group Secretariat, The Welsh Office, Cathays Park, Cardiff, CF1 3NQ, Wales.

3. *Scotland:* Scottish Home and Health Department, St Andrew's House, Regent Road, Edinburgh, EH1 3DE, Scotland.

4. *Northern Ireland:* Department of Health, Dundonald House, Upper Newtownards Road, Belfast, BT4 3SF, Northern Ireland.

British Medical Institutes

— *Cancer Research:* The Dean, The Institute of Cancer Research, McElwain Laboratories, 15 Cotswold Road, Belmont, Sutton, Surrey, SM2 5NG, UK.

— *Child Health:* The Dean, Institute of Child Health, 30 Guilford Street, London, WC1N 1EH, UK.

— *Dental Surgery:* The Dean, Institute of Dental Surgery, 256 Gray's Inn Road, London, WC1X 8LD, UK.

— *Dermatology:* The Dean The St. John's Institute of Dermatology, Block 7, St Thomas' Hospital, Lambeth Palace Road, London, SE1 7EH, UK.

— *Heart and Lung:* National Heart and Lung Institute, Dovehouse Street, London, SW3 6LY, UK.

— *Laryngology and Otology:* The Dean, Institute of Laryngology and Otology, 330–332 Gray's Inn Road, London, WC1X 8EE, UK.

— *Neurology:* The Dean, Institute of Neurology, The National Hospital, Queen Square, London, WC1N 3BG, UK.

— *Obstetrics and Gynaecology:* The Dean, Institute of Obstetrics and Gynaecology, Queen Charlotte's Hospital for Women, Goldhawk Road, London, W6 0XG, UK.

— *Ophthalmology:* The Dean, The Institute of Ophthalmology, 11–43 Bath Street, London, EC1V 9EL, UK.

— *Orthopaedics:* The Professor of Orthopaedics, The Institute of Orthopaedics, Royal National Orthopaedic Hospital, Brockley Hill, Stanmore, Middlesex. HA7 4LP, UK.

— *Psychiatry:* The Dean, Institute of Psychiatry, De Crespigny Park, Denmark Hill, London, SE5 8AF, UK.

— *Surgery:* The Raven Department of Education, Royal College of Surgeons of England, Lincoln's Inn Fields. London, WC2A 3PN, UK.

— *Tropical medicine*: Liverpool School of Tropical Medicine: The Dean, Liverpool School of Tropical Medicine, Pembroke Place, Liverpool, L3 5QA, UK.
London School of Hygiene and Tropical Medicine: Keppel Street, London, WC1, UK.

— *Urology:* The Dean, Institute of Urology, 48 Riding House Street, London, W1P 7PN, UK.

Royal Colleges

— Royal College of Anaesthetists: 48–49 Russell Square. London, WC1B 4JY, UK.
— Royal College of General Practitioners: The Secretary, Royal College of General Practitioners, 14 Princes Gate, London, SW7 1PU, UK.
— Royal College of Obstetricians and Gynaecologists: The Secretary, Royal College of Obstetricians and Gynaecologists, 27 Sussex Place, Regent's Park, London, NW1 4RG, UK.
— Royal College of Ophthalmologists: 17 Cornwall Terrace, London, NW1 4QW, UK.
— Royal College of Pathologists: The Registrar, Royal College of Pathologists, 2 Carlton House Terrace, London, SW1Y 5AF, UK.
— Royal College of Physicians (Edinburgh): The Registrar, Royal College of Physicians, 9 Queen Street, Edinburgh, EH2 1JQ, UK.
— Royal College of Physicians (Ireland): Registrar, Royal College of Physicians, 6 Kildare Street, Dublin 2, Eire.
— Royal College of Physicians (London): Examinations Department, Royal College of Physicians, 11 St Andrew's Place, Regent's Park, London, NW1 4LE, UK.
— Royal College of Psychiatrists: The Secretary, Royal College of Psychiatrists, 17 Belgrave Square, London, SW1X 8PG, UK.
— Royal College of Radiologists: The Warden, Royal College of Radiologists, 38 Portland Place, London, W1N 3DG, UK.
— Royal College of Surgeons (Edinburgh): Clerk to the College, Royal College of Surgeons, Nicolson Street, Edinburgh, EH8 9DW, UK.
— Royal College of Surgeons (England): The Examinations Secretary, Royal College of Surgeons, 35–43 Lincoln's Inn Fields, London, WC2A 3PN, UK.
— Royal College of Surgeons (Ireland): The Examinations Secretary, Examinations Office, Royal College of Surgeons, St Stephen's Green, Dublin 2, Eire.

— Royal College of Physicians and Surgeons (Glasgow): The Registrar, Royal College of Physicians and Surgeons, 234–242, St Vincent Street, Glasgow, G2 5RJ, UK.

Educational Councils and Examining Boards

— Scottish Council for Postgraduate Medical Education: The Secretary, Scottish Council for Postgraduate Medical Education, 8 Queen Street, Edinburgh, EH2 1JE, UK.
— United Examining Board, Apothecaries Hall, Blackfriars Lane, London, EC4V 6EJ, UK.

Letter writing

4

GENERAL GUIDELINES

Letters are of two kinds: business and private. The second type is obviously easier to write but there are, nevertheless, certain basic rules to be remembered:

The envelope

a. It is not a British practice to put the sender's name and address on the back of the envelope. Most British people throw away envelopes as soon as letters are opened so if you want an answer, you *must* write your full address on the letter itself.

b. It is correct to address a man as, for example, Mr J Pinter. So a qualified surgeon would be addressed on the envelope as:

> Mr Robert Turner FRCS

If the man has any other title, that should be used:

> Dr Peter Cummings MRCP
>
> Sir Thomas Walker Bt MD FRCOG

c. Letters signifying civil, military or academic honours follow the name in that order.

d. When writing a business letter to a college, a company, an hotel, a newspaper, etc., the letter must be addressed to someone. You would, in fact, write to the Principal of a college, to the Secretary or Manager of a company, to the Manager or Receptionist of an hotel and to the Editor of a newspaper.

e. A married woman or a widow is normally addressed as Mrs unless she has some other title.

f. An unmarried woman is normally addressed as Miss.

g. The word Ms is often used when the marital status of a woman is not known. Some women prefer this title.

h. There is a growing tendency to omit the title completely and simply use the name, (e.g.) Peter Brook or Peggy Fisher on the envelope.

i. The address follows the name in this order:

    i. Number of house ⎫ *on same line*
   ii. Name of street ⎭

  iii. Town or village ⎫ *on same line*
  iv. Postal code ⎭

   v. County

  vi. Country (if written from abroad), e.g.,

      Dr John Turner MB CHB DPM
      36 Pilkington Avenue
      Wakefield WF2 9DG
      West Yorkshire UK

As can be seen from the above examples, modern practice is to omit punctuation for the details of the name and address. On typewritten letters, indentation is no longer used.

The letter

a. The sender's address is written *in full* at the top right-hand side of the paper. It is not customary to put the name there. In hospitals and other places where official writing paper is printed, the address is either on the right-hand side or in the centre.

b. The date is usually written below the address: day, month, year, e.g. 7 June 2000. In private letters the date is often written, e.g., 23.3.2000.

c. In a business letter, the name and address of the person to whom the letter is written are placed on the left-hand side, at the top.

d. When one writes to an unknown person the letter begins. 'Dear Sir', or 'Dear Madam', if it is to a woman. If unsure write 'Dear Sir/Madam'.

e. When one has met the person or corresponded for some time, the name is used and the letter begins, e.g., 'Dear Dr Turner'.

f. When writing to a friend, one begins 'Dear John', 'Dear Mary' or often 'My dear Elizabeth', to a closer friend.

g. If the letter begins 'Dear Sir or Madam', the ending should be 'Yours faithfully'.

h. If the letter begins, 'Dear Miss Steele' or some other name in a semi-business correspondence, the ending should be 'Yours sincerely'.

i. 'With best wishes', 'With kindest regards' or 'Yours' are quite usual endings for letters to friends.

j. Phrases such as 'I remain your humble servant' and 'Yours respectfully' are no longer used. Nor is it British practice to use very flowery, effusive language in a letter. Write clearly and simply and briefly in a business letter.

k. Each new subject or aspect of the subject should be dealt with in a separate paragraph. Paragraphs are marked by starting a little distance from the left side, or by leaving space between the paragraphs (commonly done by typists).

MISCELLANEOUS LETTERS

Here are some examples of letters which the overseas doctor may need to write. The addresses of London hospitals are correct but the names of other places in Britain and doctors are imaginary.

It is *important to print your name in block letters* underneath your signature as foreign names are often very difficult to read in handwriting. Also notice that the British write the numbers one and seven thus: 1, 7. Figures written in the style used in continental European countries may cause delay, and even loss, to correspondence.

1. **You are writing from your own country for a place on a course in England.**

62 El Bousiry Street
El Bakry
CAIRO
Egypt

17 September 1999

The Course Organiser
Academic Centre
Whittington Hospital
London
N19

Dear Sir/Madam

I should be most grateful if you would send me the course application form for the MRCP Part 2 course in February 2000. Could you also please send me details of accommodation available near the hospital?

Yours faithfully

Omar Elayet (Dr)

2. **You are writing from your own country for a clinical attachment in England.**

> Calle Jose Caballero 24
> MADRID 7
> SPAIN
>
> 1 November 2001
>
> The Clinical Tutor
> Postgraduate Centre
> Leeds General Infirmary
> Leeds 1
>
> Dear Sir
>
> I wish to come to the UK for further study and should be grateful if you would offer me a clinical attachment in paediatrics. I enclose my CV and two references.
>
> Yours faithfully
>
> Juanita Sanchez (Dr)

3. **You are writing to an hotel in England to reserve a room.**

Tokyo Medical College
53–1, Kashiwagi
Shinjuku-Ku
Tokyo
Japan

4 July 2000

The Receptionist
Ascot Hotel
11 Craven Road
London W2

Dear Madam

I should be most grateful if you would reserve me a single room (with bathroom if possible) from 9–20 October inclusive. Please confirm the booking and tell me your terms.*

Yours faithfully

Kiyoshi Suzuki (Professor)

---

*Terms means price of room and food.

4. **You are writing for permission to visit a scientific department.**

Department of Anaesthetics
The Hammersmith Hospital
Du Cane Road
London W12 ONN

21 November 2001

Dr S Buckley FFARCS
Department of Anaesthetics
The Radcliffe Infirmary
Oxford

Dear Sir

I have been working in the above department for six months whilst on leave from my hospital in India. I should be most grateful if you would allow me to visit your department in order to see the work that is being done there. I could come at any time convenient to you.

Yours faithfully

Rao Singh (Dr)

5. **You are writing to thank someone for having allowed you to visit a department.**

Department of Cardiology
Guy's Hospital
London SE1 9RT

21 December 1999

Professor C Hocks
Department of Cardiology
St Thomas' Hospital
London SE1, 7EH

Dear Professor Hocks

Thank you so much for allowing me to visit your department and to watch some open-heart surgery being performed. It was most interesting to me.

I wonder if you would be so kind as to send me a copy of your reprint: Hocks, C.: Open-heart surgery, Surgery, 26, 4, 1998?

Yours sincerely

Hussain Ismail (Dr)

6. You are submitting a paper for publication.

Department of Medicine
St Mary's Hospital
Praed Street
London W12 INY

4 November 2000

The Editor
British Medical Journal
BMA House
Tavistock Square
WC1H 9JP

Dear Sir

I wish to submit the enclosed article for consideration for publication.

Yours faithfully

Naeem Raza (Dr)

7. You wish to take out a subscription to a journal.

Biskopshavn 17
Bergen
Norway

12 January 1999

The Subscription Manager
British Medical Journal
BMA House
Tavistock Square
WC1H 9JP

Dear Sir

I wish to take out a subscription to the British Medical Journal and enclose a cheque for the required amount. Would you please send copies to me at the above address?

Yours faithfully

Inger V Pedersen (Dr)

8. **You are writing a letter of thanks to people who have entertained you in their home.**

> 45 Grassington Avenue
> Hampstead
> London NW3
>
> 30 October 2002
>
> Dear Mr and Mrs Pulter
>
> Thank you so much for a most enjoyable evening in your home last Saturday. My wife and I appreciated your kindness very much and we look forward to welcoming you in our home when you visit Athens next Spring.
>
> With best wishes to you both
>
> Yours
>
> Costas and Helen Dafnis

9. **You are in general practice and are referring a patient to hospital.**

Some GPs write letters as in the example below. Others complete special forms provided by local hospitals. With the advent of computers and word processors, letters will become highly standardised and computerised. It is important to state the full name and sex of the patient, date of birth, address and presenting symptoms. With non-English names, it is helpful to underline the family name (surname). If the patient has been to that particular hospital before, it is useful to mention it and give the patient's hospital number if known.

47 Elm Terrace
London N14

4 December 1999

Consultant Physician
The Royal Free Hospital.
Pond Street
London NW3 20G

Dear Dr Hill

Re: Charles Oxley 26 3 42(m), 42 Liverpool Way, N14
This man has c/o backache on and off for two years. Recently he has also complained of vague discomfort in the left side of his abdomen. This is not related to food intake. Micturition and bowels normal. OE limitation of movements of spine. Abdomen NAD. Perhaps the abdomen pain originates in the spinal column and I should appreciate your opinion of him.

Yours sincerely

Michael Apostopolous (Dr)

10. **The hospital doctor must reply to the GP's letter after seeing the patient.**[*]

The following information is usually included:

1. patient's name, age, sex, address;
2. presenting symptoms (to remind the GP, who has over a thousand patients);
3. any further information gained from taking the case history;
4. findings from physical examination;
5. tests required;

---

[*]Examples of letters from hospital doctors to GPs follow some of the case histories in Chapter 5, pages 66, 98, 105, 118, and 136.

6. provisional/firm diagnosis;
7. treatment required:
    i. none
    ii. medical: drugs supplied – strength, dosage, amount
    iii. hospitalisation
    iv. surgical
    v. psychiatric;
8. prognosis;
9. what information you have given patient;
10. keep contact open and future arrangements.

11. Problem lists.

Doctors are being encouraged to start their letters with a list of a patient's medical and social problems. This encourages doctors to think holistically about their patients and means that minor problems are less likely to be forgotten. For example;

Problems:

Poorly controlled asthma Passive smoker Father unemployed Damp flat.

12. Letter from Consultant Physician to GP.

Department of Medicine
St Luke's Hospital
Cheltenham

4 May 1999

Dr R Graves
16 Fosseway
Cheltenham

Dear Doctor Graves

Mr T Baxter 3 10 69 (m), 10 Victoria Crescent, Cheltenham

After failing to keep several follow-up appointments, your

cont'd

patient came to see me this week, having finished the steroids for his ileocolonic Crohn's disease 3 weeks ago. He has regained 8.6 kg in weight and says he is now back to normal and eating well. He still gets occasional abdominal pain, and says he has had a persistent cold for the last few weeks. He is off all medication, and looking for a job after 18 months as a painter.

I could not find any significant signs on examination, apart from slight tenderness in the right lower quadrant but no mass was palpable.

His recent investigations show normal haemoglobin, with a slightly raised white count of 13.3 (10.01 neutrophils), and an ESR of 30 (1–15). His albumin has risen from the pre-treatment level of 16 to 36, and his alk. phos. has fallen from 205 to 124 (30–100). The rest of his biochemical tests are normal. The recent small bowel enema confirmed the terminal ileal disease but did not show any abnormalities higher up.

I have emphasised to him and his mother, who accompanied him, the importance of regular follow-up.

I will see him again in 2 months' time.

Yours sincerely

Henry Simmons
Consultant Physician

13. Letter from Consultant Physician to Consultant Psychogeriatrician.

Department of Gastroenterology
Queen Elizabeth Hospital
Birmingham

28 February 2001

Dr Kenneth Sawyers
Consultant Psychogeriatrician

Dear Kenneth

Mrs M Calthorpe 5 10 1919, 4 Judd Street, Birmingham
I should be grateful if you would arrange an appointment for the above patient. She is shortly returning to Glasgow so I would be grateful if you could see her fairly soon.

As you will see from her notes, she was admitted in December 1996 with small bowel obstruction, attributed to adhesions from a previous cholecystectomy, appendicectomy and Caesarian section. At the time of this acute illness, she was noted by her daughter and the doctors to be confused, but this seemed to resolve as she improved. I saw her last Spring when she had left-sided pain in the abdomen, which was probably related to the diverticular disease we subsequently demonstrated and this has not been a problem any more. She returned to an independent existence in Glasgow but when she came to visit her daughter a month ago was noted again to be increasingly forgetful. This seemed to be worse when tired in the evenings. She has always been an early waker at 5 am, rising at 7 30 am. She denies depression, and does not seem as concerned by her symptoms as her daughter. She is able to read and can remember the contents of the page when she gets to the end of it. However, she did get the date wrong on Tuesday, 27 February when she said it was 24 February 1998. I

cont'd

should add that she has been on thyroxine 100 mcg for some years and that her free T_3 was checked and found to be normal recently, as were her haemoglobin, white count, urea, electrolytes, calcium and liver function tests.

I think she probably accepts that this is a manifestation of her age of 82, but the intermittent nature of her symptoms prompted me to suggest that she should consult you.

With many thanks

Yours sincerely

George Webster
Consultant Physician

APPLYING FOR A POST

The advertisements for medical posts usually tell you to send for a job description and an application form. This you complete and it is common practice to send a typed curriculum vitae in addition because there is often not enough space on the application form for all you wish to say. Some university posts demand up to eight copies of applications so it is usual for them to be typed and sent with a covering letter.

All posts demand either testimonials or references. A testimonial is a certificate of character, conduct and qualifications and it is important to send *copies* of your testimonials and not the original, as you may need them again. It is wise to bring testimonials (in English if possible) with you when you come to England in order to save time.

Very often, however, the name and address of two or three *referees* are asked for; that means people you have worked with in recent times who will be willing to send a confidential reference on you to the hospital if required. Having chosen the people to ask, you must have their permission to give their name *before* sending in your application.

Examples of these letters follow.

1. You are asking for an application form for a post.

> 5 Margery Terrace
> Durham DH1 26Q
>
> 28 June 2002
>
> The Medical Staffing Officer
> Cheltenham General Hospital
> Cheltenham
> GL53 7AN
>
> Dear Sir/Madam
>
> I should be most grateful if you would send me an application form for the post of Registrar in the Department of Paediatrics as advertised in the British Medical Journal of 27th June.
>
> Yours faithfully
>
> N Khan (Dr)

2. You are asking for permission to use someone's name as a referee.

Department of Neurosurgery
Whittington Hospital
Highgate Hill
London N19

2 December 1999

A B Whitehouse FRCS
Department of Neurosurgery
Royal Hospital
Glasgow

Dear Mr Whitehouse

I am applying for the post of Specialist Registrar at the above hospital where I have been working for the past three months. I should be most grateful if you would allow me to use your name as a referee.

Yours sincerely

Manlio Guidetti (Dr)

3. **You are applying for a post in a hospital which does not supply application forms.** You compose the following application (the Latin words, curriculum vitae, are used).

CURRICULUM VITAE

NAME:	Surname: Khan Forename: Naeem
DATE OF BIRTH:	5th July 1970
NATIONALITY:	Pakistani
MARITAL STATUS/SEX:	Single/Male
PERMANENT ADDRESS:	27 St Albans Road, London
	SW17 5TZ
	Telephone: 0181–734 6723
MEDICAL SCHOOL:	Nishtar Medical College,
	Multan, Pakistan
GMC REGISTRATION:	Limited Registration No. 83/0542
QUALIFICATION:	MB BS – June 1996

POSTS HELD:

From	To	Post	Speciality	Hospital	Consultants
8 6 96	5 12 96	HO	Paediatric Medicine	Nishtar Hospital, MULTAN	Professor of Paediatric Medicine
6 12 96	7 6 97	HO	General Surgery	Nishtar Hospital, MULTAN	Professor of Surgery
17 6 97	16 3 98	SHO	Paediatric Medicine	Nishtar Hospital, MULTAN	Professor of Paediatric Medicine
17 3 98	28 2 99	Demon-strator	Physiology	Nishtar Medical College, MUTAN	Professor of Physiology
21 7 99	31 7 99	Locum SHO	Paediatrics	Brook General Hospital, London	Consultant Paediatrician

cont'd

5 9 99	18 9 99	Locum SHO	Paediatrics	District General Hospital, Barnsley	Consultant Paediatrician

REFEREES:* 1. Consultant Paediatrician, Brook General Hospital London SE18 4LW

2. Professor of Paediatric Medicine, Nishtar Hospital, Multan.

EXPERIENCE: Nishtar Hospital is a 1000 bedded hospital attached to Nishtar Medical College. The Department of Paediatric Medicine consists of 60 beds including neonatology section. During my job in the paediatric unit I was responsible for emergency duties in patient care and side-room laboratory work. I learnt the routine management of common paediatric problems. I was involved in undergraduate clinical teaching. During my job in the Department of Surgery I assisted in a variety of major operations and had a chance to do minor surgical procedures.

PUBLICATIONS: I reviewed all the cases of children admitted to the unit with hepatitis and presented my findings to the Journal of the Nishtar Medical College.

FUTURE PLANS: I want to obtain the MRCPCH. After my membership I will go back to Pakistan to practise in one of the Teaching Centres.

---

*One would normally give the names of the referees.

4. **The accompanying letter, which we call a 'covering letter'.**

62 Coverdale Crescent
London NW3

26 October 1999

The Medical Staffing Officer,
Whittington Hospital
Highgate Hill
London N19

Dear Sir/Madam

I wish to apply for the post of Specialist Registrar in Child Psychiatry as advertised in the British Medical Journal of 23 October.

I enclose my curriculum vitae and the names, addresses and telephone numbers of three referees as requested.

Yours faithfully,

Omar Massoud (Dr)

5. You have been offered a post but wish to postpone the commencement of duties.

42 Brook Lane
Leeds 4

5 March 2002

The Medical Staffing Officer
Leeds General Infirmary
Leeds 1

Dear Sir

Thank you for your letter of 3 March 2002 offering me the post of Senior House Officer in Medicine from 23 March 2002.

I am very pleased to accept the post but just after the interview on 1 March I received a call from my family telling me that my father had died suddenly and my mother is ill. As the eldest son of the family it is necessary for me to return to Pakistan to see the situation for myself and make necessary arrangements. Would it, therefore, be possible for you to postpone the commencement of my post to 15 April 2002 to allow me to travel to Karachi?

I should be most grateful if you would consider this, and I await your reply.

Yours faithfully

Nasir Jalil (Dr)

Communication skills for medicine

5

TALKING TO PATIENTS

Good communication between doctor and patient is vital in order to make an accurate diagnosis, to satisfy a patient and make him feel less anxious and to ensure that he follows the advice given. No medical terms should be used that the patient cannot understand. The instructions should be clear and simple. In the following outline of the different stages of taking a case history some examples of the kind of language used are given.

1. Greeting patient and introducing oneself

'Good morning, Mrs Rayner. Come and sit down. I'm Dr Adamson.'

2. Invitation to patient to describe symptoms

'Well now, how can I help you?'

or

'Well, Mrs Rayner, what's the trouble?'

These two openings are commonly used by some doctors. Others refer to the GP's letter and say, for example:

'Your doctor says you've been having trouble with your back. Tell me about it.'

3. Taking of history

Examples of language used in a systems review are on pages 167–184 and in case histories on pages 57–166. In the case histories it can be seen that the language is simple and does not include medical terms.

4. Instructions for undressing for clinical examination

Be specific. If you wish to do a thorough physical examination it is usual to say:

> 'Would you mind taking off all your clothes except your pants' (for men) 'except your pants and bra' (for women). Lie on the couch and cover yourself with the blanket' (or whatever your particular hospital provides).

Otherwise you might say, for example:

> 'Slip off your shoes and socks' (for examination of feet of men or children).
> 'Roll your sleeve up' (for examination of elbow or lower arm).

It is essential that you learn the names of garments worn by your patients.

5. Instructions for position on couch and during clinical examination

It is no use asking your patient to lie in the prone position. He will not generally understand this term. Say instead:

> 'Please lie on your tummy.'

Other examples of instructions for position are:

> 'Please turn over and lie on your back.'
> 'Roll over onto your left/right side.'
> 'Bend your knees.'
> 'Sit up.'
> 'Lean forward.'
> 'Get off the couch and stand up.'
> 'Walk across the room.'

During the clinical examination you may wish to examine certain parts of the body by instrument and you must prepare your patient for this. Doctors often use the words 'I'm going to/I'm just going to' to express something about to happen. Here, for example, an examination by sigmoidoscope:

> 'I'm just going to have a look in your back passage to make sure everything is all right. I want you to lie on your left side with your

bottom right over the edge of the couch. I'm going to examine you with my finger and then with an instrument which will feel like my finger only cold. Let yourself go loose. Try and relax. This will feel cold. Take a deep breath in. This will feel rather like the last one. Breathe in again. This may make you feel as if you want to have your bowels opened, but don't worry, you won't. I'm just going to blow some air in now. Good. I've almost finished. Good.'

Notice the constant reassurance the doctor gives by the use of 'just', 'don't worry' and 'good'.

Here is another example of a vaginal examination followed by a cervical smear test:

'I just want to have a look down below. Lie on your back with your knees bent and your legs wide apart. Good. Now try to relax. I'm just going to feel inside. Fine. Now I'm going to pass an instrument with a light to enable me to see better. It may feel cold but it won't harm you. That seems all right. Now I want to do a cervical smear test. I shall just take a specimen with this swab. Good. We'll send that off to the lab. Fine.'

6. Instruction to dress

Do not walk out of the room leaving your patient unsure of what to do next.

'You can get dressed now and then come out to me' is helpful. For a disabled or elderly patient who finds dressing difficult, it is kind to add: 'Don't hurry. Take your time.'

7. Giving information

Wait until the patient is fully dressed and out of the cubicle before giving information.

a. No treatment

Sometimes it is possible for the hospital doctor to make an immediate diagnosis and reassure the patient at once:

'Well, Mrs Turner, there doesn't seem to be anything wrong with you. I'm sure this will clear up on its own but if you continue to be worried about it, go to your GP and he will arrange for you to come and see me again.'

b. Tests

Much more often, the hospital doctor will order tests.

'Well, Miss Hartley, I can't find anything seriously wrong with you but I'd like you to have your chest X-rayed and an EEG. Take these forms to the Appointments desk before you leave the hospital.'

Most patients want to know what the tests involve. Here is an example of the actual words you may use to a patient who has to have a brain scan:

'You will be asked to lie on a couch. The couch will move through a shallow tunnel. You will be able to see on either side and nothing will touch you. The X-ray machine is fitted inside the tunnel and it takes individual pictures of different parts of the head rather like the slices of a loaf of bread. No special preparation is needed for this procedure. The radiographer may put a headband on your head to position you but you will not feel restricted. The radiographers can see you and speak to you but they will not actually be in the same room. It will only take about fifteen minutes and you will then be able to go home.'

c. Drugs

As it will usually be some time before the results of the tests are available, the doctor will prescribe drugs if necessary.

'I'd like you to have an X-ray of your shoulder and neck. I'll give you a prescription for some tablets to ease the pain.'

Your letter to the GP will notify him of the drugs prescribed.

d. Hospitalisation

It is sometimes necessary to bring the patient into hospital for specific tests. This is particularly true of children and the elderly. Words are chosen to avoid alarming the patient and the patient's relative:

'I'd like you to come / I'd like Johnnie to come into hospital for a night to find out what exactly is causing this trouble.'

e. Surgery

There are, of course, conditions which can only be dealt with by surgery:

> 'Well, Mr Green, you've had this trouble for months. We've tried tablets without any success so now I'm going to refer you to the surgeon to arrange for you to have an operation.'

Here is an example of a 76-year-old man with a gangrenous leg who needs an amputation:

> 'Well, Mr Fox, we've been trying to treat this leg with drugs but, as you can see, it hasn't responded to treatment at all. We can't let this go on any longer, because the gangrene will spread and your life could be at risk. So I'm afraid we now have no alternative but to amputate your leg below the knee. I know this is bad news for you but after your operation, once the wound has healed, we shall send you to a specialist unit where they will fit you with an artificial limb. Then we shall teach you to walk with it. You will meet people who have had the same operation and are now mobile and active again.'

f. Psychiatry

There are patients who are referred to hospital by their GPs and, after countless tests, nothing is found to be wrong. In spite of being reassured the patients still return to the hospital complaining of the same symptoms. At some point, the physician may decide to refer a patient to a psychiatrist:

> 'Well, Mrs Barnes, we've done all the necessary tests and can't find anything wrong with you but I know you still feel unwell so I'm going to refer you to a psychiatrist and hope he can help you.'

g. Imparting bad news

It is sometimes necessary to give news to the patient that is unwelcome, frightening, bad. The trend to openness means that the choice of words is extremely important in order to give the patient the information he needs to have and at the same time causing him the least anxiety possible. The phrase *I'm afraid* is commonly used to signal bad news and to express regret.

'I'm afraid this is a serious condition. You'll need an operation.'

'I'm afraid the lump is a breast cancer, so we must now talk about the best way of dealing with it.'

'I'm afraid your mother died during the operation. Her heart wasn't strong enough…'

It is helpful to a patient if a doctor shows understanding.

'I know this is bad news for you but there is a lot we can do to help you.'

b. Reassurance

All patients need reassuring whether their complaint is trivial or life-threatening. It is a complex subject and is not limited to verbal communication. The physical presence of a doctor can reassure: his appearance, manner, attitude and intonation all play a part. In spite of the complexities of the subject, certain verbal patterns of reassurance are common:

'Don't worry about this. It's quite a common condition and should clear up in a week or so.'

'This is not a serious condition. These tablets should help.'

'The only way to treat this is by an operation. It is routine surgery, we have a team of experienced surgeons here and you should be back to normal two months after the operation.'

It is important that a doctor stresses the positive aspect of a patient's condition and that the patient realises that whatever happens he can rely on the doctor's support. In life-threatening illnesses, the reassurance the doctor can give is to be near in times of crisis:

'You will no doubt want to go home as soon as possible but we are here to help you whenever you need us.'

It is now recognised that it is quite difficult for patients under stress to take in a lot of information. Doctors often use drawings to make a point of information clearer, for example to explain a hiatus hernia. Many hospitals produce information sheets and cassettes with explanations of necessary procedures and operations. The patient can study these at home. An example of part of a detailed leaflet explaining a barium enema is printed here to illustrate the simplicity of the language used, avoiding medical terms. Instructions for the time of the procedure and preparations necessary would also be provided.

THE DEPARTMENT OF IMAGING
Whittington Hospital
London N19 5NF

Barium enema information sheet

What is a barium enema?

This is an X-ray examination of your large bowel. It is performed in the X-ray department.

What preparation do you need for your barium enema?

For this examination to be successful your bowel must be as empty as possible. As part of your preparation you will be given a laxative. You will need to stay near to a toilet after taking the laxative. You need to drink plenty of fluids to avoid dehydration.

It is very important to follow instructions on eating and drinking, carefully. See the attached leaflet.

Please check whether you have a morning appointment or an afternoon appointment.

You can continue to take any medicines or pills as normal, except iron pills or medicines that make you constipated, e.g. codeine phosphate.

On the day of your barium enema

— Please come into the main X-ray department in Outpatients in good time for your appointment.

— If you arrive more than 15 minutes late you may have to rebook to avoid delaying other patients.

— The staff are very familiar with this examination and will assist you throughout. Please ask them any questions about the procedure that you may have.

— It can be a rather uncomfortable procedure but it is not usually painful.

— You lie on your side, and a small tube is inserted into your back passage and some barium (which is a thick white liquid) is fed through the tube. The barium shows up on X-ray.

— The bowel is then slightly distended with air so that the bowel lining can be seen more clearly. Then X-rays are taken of the large bowel.

— The actual procedure takes about 30 mins, but you will need to be in the department for approximately 2 hours.

— You will need to go to the toilet before and after the procedure. There is a toilet in the department.

— You may be given an injection to relax the bowel which often makes the procedure more comfortable. This injection may also cause slightly blurred vision. This is temporary and will return to normal.

After the barium enema

Please ask a friend or a relative to accompany you home.

You may return to your normal diet immediately. Your stools will appear white and may be harder than normal; this will return to normal within 2 days. To avoid constipation after the examination drink plenty of fluids and eat foods such as fruit to clear the bowel (unless your doctor specifically advises against this).

The results of your examination will be sent to the doctor who arranged for this examination within 10 days.

Important, please inform the department in advance if

1. there is any possibility that you suffer from glaucoma.
2. there is any chance that you may be pregnant.

Also please note

1. If you take oral contraceptives, they may be made ineffective by taking the laxative during your preparation. Please continue to take the oral contraceptives but use extra precautions for the rest of the cycle.
2. If you are a diabetic please continue taking your medication (insulin or tablets) during your preparation, checking your blood glucose frequently and adjusting your insulin and sugar intake accordingly.

3. If you are given the injection to relax the bowel it is important not to drive or operate machinery for at least 2 hours.

CASE HISTORIES

The following case histories are nearly all actual ones but, for reasons of confidentiality, the names of the patients have been omitted or changed. The histories come from various branches of medicine so that the kind of language used by doctors and patients can be studied. Notice the simple language used by the doctor and the avoidance of medical terminology. Patients and doctors often use colloquial expressions, and explanations of these are given. Abbreviations used will be found in full in Chapter 11.

1. Family and social history

When taking a history, it is quite often necessary to enquire about the background of the patient and to put the illness into the context of the patient's daily life and to be aware of its effect on the patient and the family.

The following questions are to help you to develop your communication skills in what is often a sensitive area requiring careful use of language. Naturally, you would use a *selection of these relevant to the particular patient.*

Family history

In Western European countries nowadays many people form stable relationships without being married. In the UK there is a high divorce rate and many people have serious relationships with someone of the same gender.

> How old are you?
> Have you got a partner?
> How long have you been together?
> Have you any children?
> How old are they?

Are they still living at home?
Are your parents alive?
How old was your father when he died?
What did he die of?
How old is your mother?
Is she well?
Have you any brothers and sisters?
How old are they?
Are they well?
Where do you come in the family?
Has anyone in your family had heart trouble, diabetes,…?

Social history

Employment

What do you do? (This means what is your work?)
Do you work full time or part time?
Do you work shifts? (This relates to irregular hours, e.g. in a factory.)
How long have you had this job?
Are you happy at work?
Do you feel under stress at work?
What did you do before this job?
How long were you in that job?
How long have you been out of work?

Accommodation

Do you live in a house / a flat / a room?
Is it your own house or do you rent it?
Do you have good neighbours?

Life style

How do you spend your free time?
Do you take any exercise?
Do you play any sports?
Have you any hobbies?
Do you go abroad for holidays?

When did you last go abroad and where?
How many hours a week do you watch TV?

Smoking history

Do you smoke?
What do you smoke?
How many cigarettes do you smoke a day?
When did you start smoking?
When did you give up smoking?
Does your partner smoke?

Drinking history
See page 178 for questions.

How much do you drink a week?
Do you know how many units?

A unit is 10 g of alcohol and this is half a pint of beer or one glass of wine or one measure of spirits. The recommended levels are 14–21 units for a woman and 21–28 units for a man spread over one week.

Drug history

1. *Prescribed*

Has your doctor prescribed any tablets for your condition?
Has any doctor prescribed you any tablets recently?

2. *OTC (over the counter)*

Are you taking any tablets of any kind that you bought from the chemist's?

3. *Recreational*

Have you tried any drugs, like cannabis?
Have you ever taken ecstasy or any hard drugs?

Stress

Do you ever feel under stress?
What sort of things make you stressed?

Tell me how you feel when you are stressed.

What do you do to relieve it?

Anxiety

Are you worried about anything?

Do certain things make you feel anxious?

Have you any money worries?

Does worry make your symptoms worse?

Sexual history

When did you first have sex?

Are you sexually active now?

Do you have a regular partner?

Have you had sex with anyone other than your regular partner?

Was this with a man or woman or both?

When you had intercourse was this vaginal or anal?

Do you have oral sex?

Heterosexual: Do you use any form of contraception?

Homosexual: Do you have unprotected sex?

How frequently do you have sex?

When did you last have sex?

Illnesses

Have you ever had any serious illnesses in the past?

Have you ever had an operation?

Have you ever been in hospital for any reason?

Did you have any problem with your pregnancies?

Have you ever had any accidents or injuries?

What is the problem now?

Did you have a healthy childhood?

Were you abused when you were a child?

Concluding remarks

Is there anything else you'd like to tell me?

What do you think is the matter with you?

How do you think I can help you?

2. Boy, aged 10

Asthmatic since aged 4. Brought into A and E Department at the suggestion of GP by his mother, following a severe asthmatic attack. Seen by Casualty Officer who calls in Paediatric SHO. Child is restless, audibly wheezing with rapid pulse rate.

Doctor: So, your GP suggested you brought Tony in?

Mother: Yes, we've had a very bad night. He's had hardly any sleep, wheezing, out of breath and coughing. I was really worried so I rang up Dr Cooper.

Doctor: Does he use a blue inhaler?[1]

Mother: Yes. He's had one for years.

Doctor: But it didn't help?

Mother: Not this time.

Doctor: Is his asthma normally under control?

Mother: Well, he's had it since he was four. I was worried about him going to school at the start but he seems to manage most of the time.

Doctor: Can you play games Tony?

Tony: Mmm, but I get breathless when I run.

Doctor: How many stairs can you climb without getting out of breath?

Tony: About ten. Sometimes more…

Doctor: Are you breathless late at night and early in the morning?

Tony: Yes but I sometimes wake up wheezing and it's horrible.

Doctor: Have you any animals at home?

(to mother)

Mother: No, he wanted a pet so we got him a cat but it made his condition worse so we had to give it away.

Doctor: Have you noticed if he's allergic to anything else?

Mother: Well, we try to keep dust down in the house.

Doctor: Who did you see about Tony's asthma in the first place?

Mother: We were sent to St Mary's and he had lots of tests to see what he was allergic to…

Doctor: And what were the results?

Mother: Oh, he was allergic to lots of things.

Doctor: So he was put on[2] Intal, was he?

Mother: Yes, he took that for years regularly, but a year ago his asthma got worse and our GP changed inhalers.

Doctor: Does he now use a brown inhaler?[3]

Mother: Yes, he uses it regularly.

Doctor: Is there anyone else in the family with hay fever, eczema or asthma?

Mother: Oh yes, my mother had asthma all her life. I had eczema as a child. On my husband's side several people have hay fever.

Doctor: Has Tony had any illnesses apart from asthma?

Mother: No, fortunately not. That's enough.

Doctor: Has he ever had to come into hospital before with a similar attack to today's?

Mother: Yes. They put him on steroid tablets. Another time he was rushed into Intensive Care and put on a machine to help him breathe.

Doctor: Has he a nebulising machine at home?

Mother: Yes and a peak flow meter. The asthma nurse showed us how to use it.

Doctor: What is Tony's usual peak flow rate?

Mother: Three hundred.

Doctor: And what was it today?

Mother: A hundred. He's been very restless all night and breathless. He took more and more puffs but he's just the same.

Doctor: Does anything special bring on one of these attacks?

Mother: It seems to be when he gets a cold.

Doctor: Mmm. That's very common. Well, Tony I'm going to bring you into hospital to get you sorted out.[4] All right?

Mother: Thank you doctor. That's a relief.

Explanations

1. **blue inhaler:** Salbutamol inhaler.
2. **put on:** prescribed.
3. **brown inhaler:** Beclomethasone inhaler.
4. **sorted out:** treated.

3. Man, aged 52

Doctor: Well, your main trouble is shortness of breath?

Patient: Yes.

Doctor: And you cough up sputum?

Patient: I what?[1]

Doctor: You cough up phlegm?

Patient: Yes.

Doctor: And you were a miner?

Patient: Yes, for fifteen years.

Doctor: Well, how bad is the shortness of breath?

Patient: I've got about fourteen steps to go up to bed and I've got to stop on the landing.[2] I haven't been able to work for two years. I'm lucky I have two sons to help me. I can't lift.

Doctor: How long has this shortness of breath bothered you?

Patient: For about two and a half to three years now, Doctor.

Doctor: Do your feet ever swell?

Patient: No, but they ache.

Doctor: Is everything else all right? Digestion, bowels, water?

Patient: I've got no trouble with the toilets.[3] My water does not bother me at all. I can eat: I like two meals a day with something solid at tea-time.[4]

Doctor: Yes. And do you smoke?

Patient: Yes. I've cut myself down to between ten and fifteen a day[5] but I've started smoking a pipe and I smoke about two ounces[6] of tobacco a week.

Doctor: As well as the ten to fifteen cigarettes?

Patient: Yes. I can't smoke a pipe after I've had my dinner and that's when I go back to my cigarettes.

Doctor: Your wife's at home, is she?

Patient: Yes, with my two youngest children.

Doctor: How old are they?

Patient: Twelve and thirteen.

Doctor: There's no illness in the family, is there? No TB?

Patient: No.

Doctor: Any illness you've had in the past?

Patient: Well, I've had bronchitis a time or two, especially in the winter months.

Doctor: Well, if you can have your woollie off[7] and lie down, I'll give you a check-up.

After examining the patient...

Doctor: Well, the trouble is bronchitis and the main cause of it is smoking, of course.

Patient: Do you think so?

Doctor: I'm sure of it. Now that doesn't mean that if you stop smoking it will get all right but it does mean that if you go on smoking it will get steadily worse. If you stopped smoking I would think that with average luck you would notice some improvement.

Patient: I've noticed a big improvement since I cut the cigarettes down and went on to a pipe because I don't inhale the pipe you see.

Doctor: I know. Well, this is the main thing. Now the other thing that you can be thinking about is the question of coal dust. I can just tell looking at your X-ray film that you've been a miner, so there must be a trace of coal dust there. You are perfectly free to apply for compensation to the Pneumoconiosis Medical Panel but my guess is that you probably wouldn't be accepted.

Patient: I'm not bothered about that, doctor.

Doctor: No, but we have to talk about this. If you want to have a go[8] all you do is to go to the local Department of Employment and put in a claim.

Patient: How are my lungs, Doctor?

Doctor: Not bad at all. If you hadn't got smoker's bronchitis, I don't think this would worry you at all.

Patient: I've been troubled with bronchitis ever since I was born, you know. It was an ailment that my mother had. She died of pneumonia. I've been chesty[9] all my life but apart from the breathing side of it, my lungs aren't opening – you know what I mean?

Doctor: Well, your tubes[10] are partly filled up, that's the thing, but it's not that bad. I get lots of people here much worse than you but I realise that it does interfere with your activities.

Patient: It stops me from lifting. I lift one or two things and then I'm jiggered.[11]

Doctor: Now apart from smoking, what else can you do? You have difficulty, I expect, clearing the chest in the morning?

Patient: Yes.

Doctor: Have you one of these little pressurised inhalers[12]?

Patient: No.

Doctor: Well, one of these would clear the chest in the morning. All you do is shake it and puff. One puff is usually sufficient. You must not have more than two puffs and no more for three hours. Is that clear? These are absolutely safe if you stick to[13] that dose. This would help to clear your chest and before you go up a hill you could have a puff. I'll write to your doctor about that, shall I?

Patient: Please. Thank you, Doctor.

Explanations

1. **I what?:** The patient does not understand the word 'sputum' so the doctor repeats the question using the word 'phlegm'.
2. **landing:** flat part of a staircase.
3. **toilets:** motions, stool.
4. **something solid at tea-time:** In the North of England a substantial meal is often eaten between 5 and 6 p.m. It is called 'high tea' or 'tea'.
5. **I've cut myself down to:** I've reduced the number of cigarettes I smoke.
6. **ounces:** See page xi.
7. **if you can have your woollie off:** if you will take your woollen pullover or cardigan off.
8. **to have a go:** to try.
9. **chesty:** had trouble with my chest, coughing.
10. **tubes:** lungs.
11. **jiggered:** exhausted, out of breath.
12. **pressurised inhaler:** salbutamol inhaler.
13. **stick to:** keep to.

Letter to GP from Consultant

Chest Hospital
Newbridge

20 March 1999

Dr Robert Walker
4 St Bede's Road
Newbridge

Dear Dr Walker

Samuel Lister (M) 2 7 1947, 32 Park Terrace, Newbridge
Yes, I agree with you that the patient's trouble is smoker's
bronchitis with airways obstruction. His peak expiratory flow
rate is not as bad as I thought it would be, 245, but of course it
is grossly reduced. The chest X-ray film shows minimal dust
change which, in my opinion, is not sufficient to qualify him as a
case of pneumoconiosis. There is, of course, no objection to his
putting in a claim.

Mr Lister can expect slow deterioration in his breathing as long
as he continues smoking. It may help him to clear his chest in
the morning if he has a salbutamol inhaler. I have explained to
him the correct dose is one puff, repeated if necessary, and
then no more for at least three hours. Please let us know if you
would like him to be seen again in the future.

Yours sincerely

John Hamilton
Consultant Physician

4. Man, aged 22

Patient attending follow-up clinic for result of his investigations. Two years previously in hospital for three weeks with duodenal ulcer symptoms. Difficult home background. Overweight. Bitten fingernails. Symptoms reappeared.

Doctor: How are you now?

Patient: Not too good.

Doctor: Are you still getting the pain?

Patient: Yes.

Doctor: Well, the X-ray doctor found irritability and distortion of the duodenum although there was no actual ulcer visible on the X-ray. This does not necessarily mean that you have no ulcer. We have to decide the best way of treating it. There are two ways: medical and surgical. In young people we try to avoid operations and we hope that medical means will help. There is no risk attached to the operation but we can't give a hundred per cent guarantee that it would relieve all your symptoms. Most patients get better after it and have no side effects. But with young people we usually persist with medical treatment. Now you did have a spell[1] in hospital and it disappeared but now it has started again. Has anyone in your family had an ulcer?

Patient: Yes, my father had one but it cleared up.[2]

Doctor: Well, this could be relevant as ulcers may run in families. But there isn't much you can do about that as you can't choose your parents! The other factors, of course, are smoking, worry, anxiety, irregular meals, over-tiredness, overwork and stress. These all affect an ulcer. Unfortunately you have a lot of stress and worry at home so I feel, despite your being so young, putting you to bed for three weeks isn't enough. I'd like you to see Mr Oakes.[3] He has a great deal of experience with ulcers and if he feels an operation is the answer, I think we should take his advice. Now, have you managed to do anything about your smoking?

Patient: I smoke about fifty a day.

Doctor: How often do you get the pain now?

Patient: Every day.

Doctor: Does it wake you up from sleep?

Patient: Once a week it does.

Doctor: Have you been sick?[4]

Patient: No.

Doctor: Have you lost time from work because of it?

Patient: Yes, odd days here and there.

Doctor: Well, make an appointment to see Mr Oakes and I'll write to him and to your doctor.

Patient: Thank you, Doctor.

Explanations

1. **a spell:** a period, a stay.
2. **cleared up:** got better, disappeared.
3. **Mr Oakes:** Fully qualified male surgeons are addressed as Mr (pronounced Mister) whereas in other branches of medicine the title is Dr (Doctor). Female surgeons are addressed as Miss or Mrs.
4. **Been sick:** vomited.

5. Woman, aged 39

Doctor: I see you've been anaemic and you had a blood test last May. Has anything else troubled you?

Patient: I've kept getting a roaring in my ears and giddiness.[1]

Doctor: Anything else?

Patient: Yes, I am breathless.

Doctor: All the time?

Patient: Most of the time.

Doctor: What do you do?[2]

Patient: I'm a cook.

Doctor: How long has all this gone on?

Patient: Say,[3] six months.

Doctor: Since your treatment with iron?[4]

Patient: Yes. I keep getting dizzy spells.[5]

Doctor: Tell me about them. How often do you get them?

Patient: They come and go but last time I fell badly.

Doctor: Does anything bring them on?

Patient: Rushing about.

Doctor: What actually happens?

Patient: I keep falling down.

Doctor: Do you know you're going to fall?

Patient: I know I'm falling but I can't stop myself.

Doctor: Do your legs give way?[6]

Patient: Yes.

Doctor: Do you fall in any particular way?[7]

Patient: I keep falling forwards.

Doctor: You've hurt yourself more than once?

Patient: Oh yes. I go giddy. The fridge comes to meet me and whizzes round.[8]

Doctor: If you stand still, do you hold on?

Patient: Yes.

Doctor: Do you feel giddy in bed?

Patient: Yes.

Doctor: Are you all right between spasms?

Patient: Yes.

Doctor: Does it affect your hearing?

Patient: I get roaring in my ears.

Doctor: What does it sound like?

Patient: Like whooshing.[9]

Doctor: How long?

Patient: Minutes.

Doctor: Do you feel sick?[10]

Patient: Yes. First thing in the morning. Terribly.

Doctor: Have you been sick?[11]

Patient: Oh yes.

Doctor: Do you suffer from headaches?

Patient: My periods[12] are only for half a day and I get terrible headaches.

Doctor: How often do you have your periods?

Patient: It varies. Every two or three weeks.

Doctor: Is it always like that?

Patient: Yes.

Doctor: When did they start?

Patient: When I was eleven. Then nine years ago they stopped for three years. I saw[13] five days before that.

Doctor: You say you are breathless?

Patient: Yes. I get puffed[14] if I go upstairs.

Doctor: Do you suffer from indigestion?

Patient: No.

Doctor: Bowel trouble?

Patient: No.

Doctor: Water?

Patient: No.

Doctor: Do you get up at night?

Patient: No.

Doctor: How's your appetite?

Patient: Fair.

Doctor: Have you lost any weight?

Patient: No.

Doctor: Do you smoke?

Patient: Fifteen to twenty a day.

Doctor: Do you drink?

Patient: Not a lot.

During the clinical examination the doctor made the following remarks:

Doctor: Can I have your arm? I'll take your blood pressure. Apart from iron tablets, are you taking anything else?

Patient: Yes. For sleeping.

Doctor: Let me look at your chest for a moment. Take a big breath. What are these pale patches on your cheeks?

Patient: They come from taking sleeping pills.

Doctor: Breathe through your mouth. When did you have your teeth out?

Patient: Four years ago.

Doctor: Let your shoulders go loose. Have your motions changed in colour?

Patient: Yes. They are very dark. The iron tablets give me diarrhoea.

Doctor: I'll look at your eyes now. Look at my finger. Keep your head still and follow it with your eyes. Open your mouth. Can you feel this pin?

I can't find any serious cause for anaemia. I'd like you to have your chest X-rayed, a skull X-ray, an EEG and some further blood tests.

Explanations

1. **roaring:** a loud noise.
   giddiness: vertigo.
2. **what do you do?:** what is your job?
3. **say:** about, roughly.
4. The doctor is seeking confirmation and expects the answer 'yes'.
5. **dizzy spells:** periods of vertigo.
6. **give way:** collapse.
7. **any particular way:** in a certain direction.
8. **the fridge ... whizzes round:** She has the impression the refrigerator is moving towards her and moving round rapidly.
9. **whooshing:** the sound of a heavy volume of water like a waterfall.
10. **feel sick:** nausea.
11. **been sick:** vomited.
12. **periods:** menstruation.
13. **I saw:** I menstruated.
14. **puffed:** out of breath, breathless.

6. Woman, aged 72

Woman complained of tightness in abdomen associated with belching wind which did not relieve feeling. Symptoms usually began between 5 and 6 p.m. lasting several hours. Relieved by white mixture.

Doctor: Does the pain come on in the night?[1]

Patient: Not often.

Doctor: When it comes on, do you get up?

Patient: Yes, I get up and walk round and it relieves it.

Doctor: Does anything but the white mixture help it?

Patient: I've been on a strict diet for six months. I never touch milk.[2]

Doctor: Does any position help you?

Patient: No, It comes on after tea, about five. I have my main meal midday.

Doctor: Have you been sick?[3]

Patient: Only at the beginning. I was very sick then.

Doctor: Do you feel sick?[4]

Patient: Yes, I feel sick but I can't be sick.

Doctor: Does the pain go through to the back?

Patient: No, but it goes under my armpits.

Doctor: What's your weight been doing?

Patient: I've lost $1\frac{1}{2}$ stone[5] but I've been on a fat-free diet for six months.

Doctor: What's your appetite like?

Patient: Poor as ever.

Doctor: What about your bowels?

Patient: I go twice a day, in the morning.

Doctor: Is this a life-long habit?

Patient: Yes.

Doctor: What do the motions[6] look like? Well-formed, firm?

Patient: Yes.

Doctor: What about the colour? Has it changed?

Patient: No.

Doctor: Are they dark?

Patient: Yes.

Doctor: Any sign of blood?

Patient: No.

Doctor: Do they float on the water when you flush the lavatory?[7]

Patient: No.

Doctor: Have you noticed an unpleasant smell?

Patient: No.

Doctor: Have you noticed any difference in your water?[8]

Patient: No.

Doctor: Do you have to get up in the night?

Patient: Once.

Doctor: Your water hasn't been darker?

Patient: No.

Doctor: Do you smoke?

Patient: Ten a day.

Doctor: Do you drink?

Patient: Not much.

Doctor: Have you any other trouble?

Patient: No, my angina's been very good.[9] I've not had much trouble with that for two years.

Doctor: You've also had trouble with your leg?

Patient: Yes, they thought it was thrombosis.

Doctor: When did you first start with your tummy trouble?[10]

Patient: About fourteen years ago.

Doctor: The same, but more bothersome now?[11]

Patient: Yes, it's tighter.

Doctor: Have you ever been jaundiced?

Patient: No.

Doctor: Is your tummy swollen when you feel like this?

Patient: It feels as though I'm going to burst.

Doctor: Well, I'd like to have a look at you. Will you get undressed and lie on the couch please?

During the clinical examination the doctor asked the following questions:

Doctor: Do you suffer from heartburn?[12]

Patient: No.

Doctor: Have you had any children?

Patient: No.

Doctor: Are your hands always cold and blue?

Patient: Yes. A lovely colour in the winter![13]

Doctor: Just hold your breath for a moment. Breathe through your mouth. Show me where you get this pain. Your age?

Patient: Seventy-two.

Doctor: Your periods finished when?

Patient: When I was about fifty-two or -three.

Doctor: Any tenderness here?

Patient: It's a bit sore[14] but not a lot.

Doctor: Does it catch you at all when you breathe?

Patient: No.

Doctor: Have you any pains in your legs?

Patient: I get cramp[15] a bit when I'm in bed.

Doctor: More in one leg than the other?

Patient: I get it in my right leg; that's my varicose leg.

Doctor: Apart from this, you've had no other serious illness in the last fourteen years?

Patient: No.

Doctor: I'm going to take a drop of your blood[16] and I'd like you to have a stomach X-ray. You'll have to come specially, don't eat anything before and drink a white paste which outlines your stomach and we'll take some pictures.[17]

Explanations

1. **come on:** start.
2. **never touch:** don't drink (or eat).
3. **been sick:** vomited.
4. **feel sick:** experience nausea.
5. **1½ stone:** See page xi.
6. **motions:** stools.
7. **flush the lavatory:** cleanse the lavatory by a flow of water.
8. **water:** urine.
9. **angina:** Angina pectoris is generally referred to as 'angina' and should not be confused with Vincent's angina (a throat condition).
10. **tummy:** stomach.
11. **bothersome:** causing trouble.

12. **heartburn:** burning sensation behind the sternum.
13. **A lovely colour:** An ironical remark. She means they are a deep blue in winter.
14. **sore:** tender.
15. **cramp:** muscle contraction.
16. **a drop of your blood:** Notice how the doctor uses 'a drop of blood' instead of 'some' to minimise the amount and therefore make the patient feel less worried.
17. **pictures:** This is a simple description of a barium meal.

7. Man aged 57

Referred by GP to Gastroenterology Clinic complaining of pain in right upper quadrant and stomach and acid reflux from stomach to gullet.

Doctor: Hello, Mr Alvarez. Come and sit down. Your doctor has sent us a letter about your problems. You've had blood in your water and chest pain. You had an ECG for that and nothing serious showed up. And now you've got pain again in your chest. And you've recently had an ultrasound scan of your abdomen?

Patient: Yes, and the result was all right.

Doctor: Yes, and you had a normal endoscopy two years ago. Well, how are you now?

Patient: My stomach always feels full up and I get a lot of pain.

Doctor: What kind of pain?

Patient: A sharp pain.

Doctor: How long have you been getting it?

Patient: A year and a half. Just the same as before.

Doctor: Have you noticed anything different?

Patient: No.

Doctor: How often do you get it?

Patient: On a good day I have no pain but on a bad day I get a lot.

Doctor: So does it come out of the blue?[1]

Patient: Yes, yesterday I had it from tea time till ten at night.

Doctor: Does it wake you up at night?

Patient: I sleep badly. I wake up because of poor breathing.

Doctor: When you get pain in the day, is it when you are hungry or after eating?

Patient: Before I eat.

Doctor: If you eat you feel better?

Patient: Yes, at first, but then it comes back again.

Doctor: How soon after?

Patient: Thirty minutes.

Doctor: Do certain foods bring on[2] pain?

Patient: Oranges and orange juice seem to be too acid.

Doctor: Do you have any problem swallowing food or liquid? Does it ever stick going down?

Patient: No.

Doctor: What happens if you drink something hot?

Patient: It burns as it goes down.[3]

Doctor: If you drink fizzy water, do you burp?[4]

Patient: Yes, and I feel better.

Doctor: Do you ever vomit?

Patient: No.

Doctor: Have you ever brought up blood?[5]

Patient: No.

Doctor: Do you bring up nasty tasting liquid?[6]

Patient: Yes, bitter and sour.

Doctor: So this has been going on for nearly two years. Are you taking any medication?

Patient: I used to take tablets for my ulcer. They were red and yellow.

Doctor: Omeprazole or Losec?

Patient: Yes, that's it.

Doctor: How often did you take Losec?

Patient: One for twenty days.

Doctor: When you took it, it worked well?[7]

Patient: Yes.

Doctor: Did you take any other tablets?

Patient: No, I used to take Rennies.[8]

Doctor: So apart from this trouble, you are otherwise well?

Patient: Yes, touch wood.[9]

Doctor: Now tell me what you do.[10]

Patient: I make sandwiches in a snack bar. I'm very busy – no time to eat in the day.

Doctor: So you have irregular meals?

Patient: Well, my wife cooks me a nice dinner at night.

Doctor: Do you drink a lot, smoke?

Patient: I never go to pubs but we have a glass of wine with our dinner. I used to smoke but I stopped two months ago.

Doctor: Did you smoke a lot?

Patient: Fifteen a day.

Doctor: Was it easy to give up[11] smoking?

Patient: Yes, I'm eating better now.

Doctor: Are the bowels all right?

Patient: Yes.

Doctor: Do you ever see any blood in your motions?[12]

Patient: No.

Doctor: You say your sleeping is sometimes affected by your breathing. Have you had any serious illnesses or operations?

Patient: No.

Doctor: Is your wife in good health?

Patient: Yes, apart from high blood pressure.

Doctor: Any children?

Patient: One boy. He's twenty-one and at University. He's very fit.

Doctor: Any brothers or sisters?

Patient: I have seven brothers and two sisters. They are all well and living in Spain.

Doctor: How about your parents?

Patient: My mother died at ninety of a heart attack and my father at seventy-seven of a stroke.[13]

Doctor: Have you any worries?

Patient: No, except about this pain. I'm worried in case it's cancer.

Doctor: We did a test to set your mind at rest.

Patient: Yes, but I still worry.

Doctor: And your doctor did a heart test and that was all right too.

Patient: I know. When I'm on holiday in Spain with my family I have no pain at all.

Doctor: Well, we all have worries. I'd like to examine you. Just go next door, slip off your trousers and shoes and lie on the couch. I'll be with you in a minute.

After clinical examination:

Doctor: Well, Mr Alvarez. I can't find anything seriously wrong with you. I'd like you to have a blood test before you leave the hospital, which I expect to be normal. I am sure you do not need to worry about cancer. Your trouble is almost certainly due to acid coming back from your stomach into your gullet[14] and irritating it. Nowadays we call this GORD which stands for Gastro Oesophageal Reflux Disease. Is there anything you want to ask me?

Patient: No.

Doctor: Well, I'll write to your doctor. There's no need for further investigation but you are always welcome to come and see me.

Patient: Thank you doctor. Goodbye.

Explanations

1. **come out of the blue:** come unexpectedly.
2. **bring on:** cause.
3. **as it goes down:** as I swallow.
4. **fizzy water:** effervescent; **burp:** bring up wind.
5. **brought up blood:** produced blood from the oesophagus.
6. **bring up nasty tasting liquid:** acid regurgitation.
7. **it worked well:** it was effective.
8. **Rennies:** over-the-counter tablets for indigestion.
9. **touch wood:** a reference to the habit of touching something wooden to avert bad luck.
10. **what you do:** what your job is.
11. **give up:** stop.
12. **motions:** stools.

13. **stroke:** cerebrovascular accident.
14. **gullet:** oesophagus.

8. Girl, aged 10½

Doctor: You're Sheila and your problem is tummy aches.[1] Tell me about them.

Patient: I mostly get them in the night. Sometimes I feel sick.[2]

Doctor: How often do you get them?

Patient: Nearly every day.

Doctor: Is it a sharp pain?

Patient: Yes.

Doctor: Do you get them before you go to bed or after?

Patient: I get them mostly when I lie down.

Doctor: Do you get them just after eating?

Patient: No.

Doctor: So you get them just after you've gone to bed usually?

Patient: Yes.

Doctor: How long do they last?

Patient: Sometimes minutes, sometimes hours.

Doctor: Are you ever actually sick?[3]

Patient: Yes.

Doctor: Do you feel better or worse after being sick?[4]

Patient: Well, my tummy feels better.

Doctor: Have you ever had this pain and sickness at school?

Patient: Yes, and I was sent home.

Doctor: How long have you been having these pains?

Patient: For two months.

Doctor: How many brothers and sisters have you?

Patient: One brother.

Doctor: How old is he?

Patient: Fifteen in December.

Doctor: Does he bully[5] or tease you – or both?

Patient: He bullies me.

Doctor: Do you like school?

Patient: No, not much (hesitantly).

Doctor: What don't you like about it? The teachers, the children or the work?

Patient: Oh, I like the teachers and the work.

Doctor: So you don't like the other children?

Patient: (Pulls a face[6] but does not answer.)

Mother: I work there serving school meals and I wonder if that had anything to do with it. At five she had terrible cramp.[7] We thought it was nerves and worry but she's been fine since. She brings up this kind of clear liquid when she's sick. Not any food.

Doctor: Does she go pale?

Mother: No. She just goes out of the room and it happens very quickly. Normally she's very lively.

Doctor: What about water?[8] Has it been more frequent?

Mother: No.

Doctor: It doesn't hurt when she goes,[9] does it?

Mother: Well, she's started to complain about that recently so I thought I'd better see the doctor about it.

Doctor: Is it when you start to pass water or at the end that it hurts?

Patient: At the end.

Doctor: Is her water quite clear?

Mother: Yes.

Doctor: Would you slip off your dress and sandals and I'll just
(to girl): have a look at your tummy.

While examining her:

Doctor: Put one finger on the spot where it hurts most. What sort of pain is it?

Patient: Like daggers.[10] Very sharp.

Doctor: When you get this pain what do you do?

Patient: I sometimes lie flat.

Doctor: What's your brother going to do when he leaves school?

Patient: I don't know.

Doctor: What does your daddy do?

Patient: He's a postman.

Doctor: He has to get up early then?[11]

Patient: Yes.

Doctor: Would you like to work in the Post Office when you leave school?

Patient: No.

Doctor: What are you best at at school?

Patient: English and Arithmetic.

Doctor: What is your favourite subject?

Patient: Geography but I'm good at English.

Doctor: Do you read much?

Patient: Yes.

Doctor: What kind of things do you read?

Patient: Sometimes murder, sometimes comics[12] and sometimes adventure.

Doctor: Quite a variety. Does it hurt down here?

Patient: Only a little pain.

Doctor: Do you get headaches with your tummy pains?

Patient: Sometimes yes, sometimes no.

Doctor: Leap down,[13] and get your clothes on. (sarcastically to mother) She's a real invalid.

Mother: Not for long. She's generally a real tomboy.[14]

Doctor: Tell me a bit more about school. About not liking it. Has it come on in the last two months?

Patient: Yes. (reluctantly) There's a boy who is nasty to me.

Doctor: How? He calls you names?

Mother: Go on. Tell Doctor about it.

Patient: He tries to put his hand up our dresses.

Doctor: Oh, that is very annoying. You'll be going to a new school in a year.

Patient: (joyfully) Yes. An all girls' school.

Doctor: Well, I can't find anything wrong with her. We'll have a blood check but I think she knows herself what is wrong. It is obviously nervous tension that is upsetting her stomach.

Girl leaves room.

Mother: I've been so worried about her. She's an odd character.[15]

She's so different in temperament from me. We are not always on the same wavelength.[16]

Doctor: That's quite common with mothers and daughters.

Mother: She's full of personality and very much on the ball[17] but she's an excitable child.

Doctor: Does she get anxious over things?

Mother: Inwardly perhaps so.

Doctor: Had she told you about this boy?

Mother: Oh yes. We'd had it all out.[18] But as Sheila is such a tomboy, I decided it was six of one and half a dozen of the other.[19] I let it go. Perhaps I shouldn't have. Then one day she got really upset and went to see the headmistress. He does it to a lot of the girls but Sheila seems to mind more than they do. She doesn't like the look of the boy.

Doctor: She is ten and a half. Does she know?[20]

Mother: Oh yes. I've told her everything. She kept asking so many questions I had to.

Doctor: Girls of this age get tummy pains. I expect all this will simmer[21] down. She's not a disturbed child. Good. Well then, nurse will arrange for the test and come and see me again in a week's time when we've got the result. But don't get too worried. I'm sure it will all clear up.

Mother: Thank you, Doctor.

Explanations

1. **tummy ache:** abdominal pain.
2. **feel sick:** nausea.
3. **are you ever actually sick?:** Do you ever vomit?
4. **after being sick:** after vomiting.
5. **bully:** use his strength to frighten or hurt.
6. **pulls a face:** grimaces.
7. **cramp:** abdominal pain of a colicky kind.
8. **water:** urine.
9. **when she goes:** when she passes water; micturates.
10. **daggers:** knife used as a weapon.

11. a statement-question, see Case History 17, note 7.
12. **comics:** magazines for children.
13. **leap down:** jump down.
14. **tomboy:** girl who likes rough, noisy games.
15. **odd character:** unusual character.
16. **not always on the same wavelength:** don't always understand one another.
17. **on the ball:** alert.
18. **had it all out:** discussed it fully.
19. **six of one and half a dozen of the other:** she was as much at fault as he was.
20. **does she know?:** does she know the facts of life?
21. **simmer down:** decrease, become less.

9. Man, aged 28

A man complains of a 4 year history of episodic headache, occurring perhaps once a month, lasting around a day, and often associated with sickness.[1]

Doctor: Do these headaches occur at any particular time?
Patient: No, they can come on at any time during the day, and sometimes they wake me.
Doctor: Tell me where the headaches are.
Patient: Usually they're at the front, and almost always on the right.
Doctor: What sort of pain is it?
Patient: It varies, sometimes it's a dull ache, but quite often it is throbbing.
Doctor: I gather[2] the headache lasts about a day?
Patient: That's correct. Sometimes, however, they have gone on[3] into the second day.
Doctor: Does anything make the headache worse?
Patient: I've noticed coughing does that, and also sneezing.
Doctor: How severe is the pain?
Patient: Sometimes it's quite mild, but at other times I have to go to bed.

Doctor: Do you feel sick with it?[4]

Patient: Usually I do, and sometimes I actually throw up.[5]

Doctor: Does the light or noise upset you?

Patient: Often both, particularly in the bad attacks.

Doctor: What pain-killers[6] help you?

Patient: It varies. Aspirin can help, but sometimes I take something stronger.

Doctor: Can anything bring the headache on?

Patient: Occasionally having a drink[7] seems to set it off,[8] particularly red wine.

Doctor: Do you get any other symptoms with it?

Patient: Perhaps twice a year, I get a pattern of zig-zag lights on my left hand side which spreads across my vision for about twenty minutes before the headaches start.

Doctor: Is your vision normally OK?[9]

Patient: Yes, its fine.

Doctor: You haven't noticed double vision, speech difficulty or problems with balance?

Patient: No.

Doctor: Do you get pins and needles[10] in the attacks?

Patient: No.

Doctor: Tell me about your general health.

Patient: It's usually good. I do get colic[11] sometimes, which my doctor says is due to an irritable colon. I used to wheeze[12] when younger, but not for years.

Doctor: Any other major illnesses in the past?

Patient: I had a road accident three years ago and broke my left leg.

Doctor: Is there any headache in the family?

Patient: My nan[13] used to have bad headaches, though they got better as she got older.

Doctor: What is your work?

Patient: I'm out of work[14] at present.

Doctor: You don't smoke or drink?

Patient: I stopped smoking three years ago – before that I smoked about twenty roll-ups[15] a day. I have about four pints[16] at the weekend.

Doctor: Could you undress down to your vest and pants please?

During the clinical examination the doctor asks the following questions:

Doctor: I notice you've got this small lump on your shoulder.
Patient: I've had that for years. The GP says it's a fatty tumour.
Doctor: Your left eyelid is lower than your right.
Patient: Yes, that seems to run in our family.
Doctor: Your blood pressure is up a bit – has that been found before?
Patient: It was at a medical[17] a year ago, but my doctor has checked it since, and it's been OK.
Doctor: Finally, can I get you to walk as if you're on a tight-rope.[18] Thank you, that's fine. Could you get dressed please?
Doctor: Your examination was fine[19] but I think it might be wise for us to arrange a scan.[20] I'm sure it will be OK but I'll drop you a line when I have the result.

Explanations

1. **sickness:** vomiting.
2. **gather:** understand.
3. **gone on:** continued.
4. **feel sick:** experience nausea.
5. **throw up:** vomit.
6. **pain-killers:** analgesics.
7. **having a drink:** usually implies alcohol.
8. **set it off:** precipitate it.
9. **OK:** normal.
10. **pins and needles:** paraesthesiae.
11. **colic:** usually refers to fluctuating abdominal pain, most often from the gut, but sometimes from other organs.
12. **wheeze:** to make an audible noise when breathing, typically in asthmatics.
13. **nan:** grandmother.

14. **out of work:** unemployed.
15. **roll-ups:** cigarettes the patient makes himself.
16. **pints:** in this context, means beer.
17. **medical:** a routine health check.
18. **tight-rope:** walking heel-to-toe.
19. **fine:** normal.
20. **scan:** in this context, either a CT or MRI scan.

10. Woman, aged 60

Diabetic, previously had bleeding ulcer treated with Zantac. Referred by GP complaining of pain all over body.

Doctor: Your GP says you're getting pain all over your body.

Patient: Yes. I was brought here by ambulance in 1968. I was in agony[1] for weeks and months. I've had a collar and a surgical corset but I'm still in pain.

Doctor: How often do you get the pain?

Patient: Every moment of the day I have pain from top to toe.

Doctor: If you had to point to one place where it is worst, where would it be?

Patient: My back. In 1972 they removed a cyst from my toe. They gave me an injection in my spine. The following day I had bleeding from down below.[2] I was in hospital one month. Since that time I've had pain in my back. I take paracetamol. They told me it was spondylitis in my neck. They gave me heat treatment and a collar. I used it for years.

Doctor: Do you have any tingling of the feet or hands?

Patient: Yes, I'm diabetic. I feel pins and needles.

Doctor: How are the waterworks?[3]

Patient: All right.

Doctor: Bowels?

Patient: All right.

Doctor: Have you had any operations?

Patient: No. Only appendix.

Doctor: When did you last have your back X-rayed?

Patient: Long ago.

Doctor: Are you taking any tablets?

Patient: I take twenty-six units of insulin for my diabetes. I have Zantac for my ulcer, tablets for my hay fever and also two glibenclamide for my diabetes.

Doctor: Who looks after your diabetes?

Patient: Dr Holman at St Mary's. I've put on so much weight.[4] They want me to go on a diet.

Doctor: Come through this way. Take off everything to your underwear. (Patient undresses.) I'm going to start off by examining your hands.

Patient: They're very painful.

Doctor: Are they worse in the morning or evening?

Patient: Morning. I do a bit of housework and I get pain.

Doctor: Are you stiff? Put your hands above your head. Good. Now behind your back. Swing your legs onto the couch. Where does it hurt? Just relax. Bend the legs. Can you feel me touching them? Do both sides feel the same? Now lie on your tummy and I'll look at your back. Roll over. I'm just going to pummel[5] your back a bit. Tell me if it hurts.

Patient: When I lie down like this the pain is so bad I grip my hands. I don't know what to do.

After the clinical examination, the patient dressed.

Doctor: Well, I'm going to get some blood tests done to see what is causing the pain in your joints. I'll also get an X-ray of your back.

Patient: They said it was osteoarthritis.

Doctor: Yes, well there is very little we can do for that. I'm going to refer you to the Pain Relief Clinic. It is run by[6] an anaesthetist. He has a lot of experience with pain and may be able to offer you advice. I'll write to your doctor and tell him I've seen you.

Explanations

1. **in agony:** in extreme pain.
2. **bleeding from down below:** vaginal bleeding.
3. **waterworks:** bladder.

4. **put on weight:** weight has increased.
5. **to pummel:** strike (usually with the fist).
6. **run by:** managed by.

11. Woman, aged 17

Insulin dependent diabetic for 10 years; she has recently been told that she has diabetic kidney disease and diabetic eye disease.

Doctor: Good morning Anna. How are you?

Patient: Good morning. I'm fine.

Doctor: Well, we didn't see you at your last appointment which was six months ago. What actually happened?

Patient: I forgot about it so I came today.

Doctor: Did you not realise that your appointment had come up?

Patient: Yes, but then something else came up at the same time and so I couldn't really come to the Clinic, so I was...

Doctor: All right. So anyway let's find out how things have been going. Tell me about your blood sugar control.

Patient: It is more or less as usual. It goes from sometimes eight to sometimes fifteen, sometimes even more than that.

Doctor: And have you been adjusting your insulin when it goes high, and do you do anything when you have low sugars?

Patient: Well, when I have gone off sugar I just eat a bar of chocolate or something, and when it is high – no, I don't do anything. I just carry on[1] the usual way.

Doctor: So you haven't been adjusting your insulin then?

Patient: Not really. Eight months ago I spoke to the nurse and she changed my morning insulin. She increased the Actrapid in the morning and she reduced the Monotard at night, and then I continued to do the same thing.

Doctor: But you are still having hypos?[2]

Patient: No. I do have high sugars sometimes at night perhaps when I forget my insulin or maybe because I have been trying to lose weight.

Doctor: You are trying to lose some weight are you? Well, how much weight have you lost?

Patient: A few kilograms.

Doctor: Well, according to my records you have lost something like eight kilograms in the last eight months which I think is probably related to your poor diabetes control and is a bit worrying.

Patient: Well, it looks good, doesn't it?

Doctor: Well, yes, it might do, but looking at your sugar today it is twenty-five and it should be between four and eight, and there are ketones in your urine which is a sign that the diabetes is very poorly controlled.

Patient: Yes, yes all right.

Doctor: Yes, but this could be potentially dangerous if you don't actually take some action about it. So I think we are going to have to increase your insulin to cover these high sugars. Do you understand that?

Patient: Oh yes.

Doctor: Right. Last time I spoke to you I told you that your kidneys had been affected by the diabetes. It is essential that we improve your control and I started you on tablets so that your kidneys would be protected from the high sugars. Have you managed to continue with that?

Patient: No, I only took the two weeks you gave me. Just two weeks of treatment.

Doctor: So for all these months then you have had no treatment?

Patient: No. No, I didn't have any.

Doctor: Well, I am sorry – there is probably some misunderstanding but you really should have gone to your GP for a prescription and continued with those tablets. They are very important to protect your kidneys. You have got a lot of protein in your urine now which is a sign that the kidneys are under stress from the diabetes.

Patient: Yes, but also I was coughing at night and I think those tablets were giving me all the troubles.

Doctor: Well yes, that is a possible side-effect, but I think you also told me that you smoke quite heavily and you do have a bit of a cough throughout the day and maybe the night-time. Is that true?

Patient: When I was here and when I smoke I do have a cough, but I think it was worsened by the tablets at the time.

Doctor: You think so; so things are better now, are they?

Patient: The cough, yes, it is better.

Doctor: Well it is a bit difficult to be sure about this, so what I shall do is to check your blood pressure and we should take some more blood today to see how your kidneys are working and we will send that to the Lab with the urine sample that you brought today, yes?

Patient: OK.

Doctor: Right. Let's go and check your blood pressure then. Oh, in fact that is quite high for you, it is 140 over 90.

Patient: Yes, OK.

Doctor: Well, it should be more like 120 over 80 or less. So it is important that we get you back on those tablets. If that cough doesn't come back then fine we will continue with it. If it does, let me know and perhaps we can change you onto a different sort of tablets. All right?

Patient: OK. Do you think that other things that I might take would affect my kidneys?

Doctor: Such as what?

Patient: Well, I drink a little bit.

Doctor: How much do you drink? How much alcohol do you drink?

Patient: When I go out at weekends I drink a pint, maybe some whisky, maybe I smoke a little cannabis.

Doctor: Well, the alcohol itself ought not to affect your kidneys. How much cannabis are you taking?

Patient: I'm not sure. We go out for a few hours. I just smoke a few.

Doctor: Well, I can't tell you that is good for you, but I don't think it is specifically doing any damage to your kidneys, but clearly this is something which I am sure you know is not good, because it is habit forming and it influences all other aspects of your life. I suggest that if you possibly can you break off that sort of habit, yes?

Patient: Yes, I can try but we enjoy it.

Doctor: We have a smoking rehabilitation nurse who you can have a chat with, and also with the diabetes specialist nurses. They can perhaps put you in touch with groups, people of your own age, you might want to discuss these sort of issues with. Would that be useful?

Patient: Yes, thank you.

Doctor: We can arrange that, but I think first of all let's get your sugar sorted out[3] and let's look at the kidney side of things. Now finally, what about your eyes. Did you go and see the ophthalmologist?

Patient: No, my next appointment is in a few months' time.

Doctor: Have you noticed any deterioration in your vision?

Patient: Maybe a little bit of blurred vision.

Doctor: Again that could be because of your high sugars. I'll put some Tropicamide drops in now. If you can wait for ten to fifteen minutes I'll look at your eyes but you must go and see the ophthalmologist anyway. All right?

Patient: OK.

Doctor: So if you take this piece of paper to the nurse she will organise all your tests, and make an appointment for four months so that I can see how you are getting on.

Patient: Four months?

Doctor: Yes, is that all right?

Patient: Well, usually it is every six months.

Doctor: Yes, but I need to see you sooner to assess your progress.

Patient: I don't know if I can because I am going on holiday.

Doctor: When?

Patient: In a month's time.

Doctor: For how long?

Patient: Well, as long as I have got money, so it could be a couple of months. We are travelling around.

Doctor: Where are you going on this holiday?

Patient: India.

Doctor: Are you going with friends or on your own?

Patient: I'm going with three friends.

Doctor: Are you taking all your needles and syringes and have you got enough information on how to get insulin? You will need a letter from a doctor to take with you about your treatment.[4]

Patient: Yes. My GP is dealing with it.

Doctor: Right. Well, I will write to your GP and I'll get all these tests organised as we discussed. I probably won't see you before you go to India so please make sure you see the nurse and I hope to see you as soon as you get back.

Patient: OK. Thanks.

Explanations

1. **carry on:** continue.
2. **hypos:** hypoglycaemic attacks.
3. **sorted out:** organised, put right.
4. **about your treatment:** a letter to show she is diabetic and needs needles and syringes for her treatment and not drug abuse.

12. Man, aged 38

Referred by GP to Outpatients complaining of loss of weight, vomiting, oedema and nocturia.

Doctor: Good morning, Mr Hartley. Come and sit down. Well now, your doctor says you've been having trouble with your water[1] for some time.

Patient: Yes, that's right. I have to keep getting up[2] in the night.

Doctor: How many times?

Patient: Oh, up to six times lately.

Doctor: Have you noticed any change in your water?

Patient: Yes, it's darker, reddish. I wonder if it could be blood.

Doctor: Have you noticed anything else?

Patient: Yes. I've been sick[3] several times in the morning and after work in the evening I've noticed my legs are puffed up.[4]

Doctor: How is your general health?

Patient: Well, I've felt really groggy[5] for some weeks now. I don't seem to enjoy my food any more and I've lost weight.

Doctor: How much?

Patient: About a stone.[6] I can tell by my clothes and my wife's worried about it. She made me go to my doctor.

Doctor: How long have you had this trouble?

Patient: About 3 months really.

Doctor: Have you ever had trouble with your water before?

Patient: Yes. A couple of years ago I had burning when I passed water. The doctor said I had high blood pressure as well and he put me on tablets and it cleared up.[7]

Doctor: Well, I'd like to examine you. Take off all your clothes except your underpants. Lie on the couch under the blanket and I'll be with you in a moment.

After examining the patient:

Doctor: You can get dressed now ... Well, Mr Hartley, I think your problem is due to the fact that the kidneys are not working as well as they should be. I want you to have some blood tests, X-rays and kidney function tests. I want you to collect your urine for twenty-four hours. Nurse will tell you exactly how to do it. Then we'll ask you to come in for an ultrasound examination of the kidneys. This is a very simple procedure to make sure there is no obstruction.

Follow-up clinic

Doctor: Hello, Mr Hartley. Come and sit down. Well, as I told you, the kidneys are not working as well as they should be. I'm going to send you to a dietitian and she will give you advice on a low-protein diet. This is not unpleasant[8] and it will lower the chemicals in your blood. It is the protein in the diet that causes a build-up of substances in the blood when the kidneys are not working normally. This makes you feel unwell. I'm also going to give you some tablets to help to keep the bones healthy. This is necessary in people with kidney disease.

Patient: Can you tell me exactly what is wrong with my kidneys?

Doctor: Well, the tests show that it is probably a condition called chronic glomerulonephritis which has damaged the kidneys. The condition is irreversible[9] – nothing can be done to put it right at this stage I'm afraid.[10] You've undoubtedly had it for a long time. We'll need to keep an eye on you.[11] There are fortunately treatments to make up for the kidney damage.

Some weeks later

Doctor: I gather[12] you've been having more trouble since I last saw you?

Patient: Oh yes. I've kept vomiting and feeling dreadful.[13] I can't keep on like this.[14]

Doctor: Mmm. Well, it looks as though the next step will be to get you into hospital to start further treatment. I think you are going to need peritoneal dialysis treatment.

Patient: What's that Doctor?

Doctor: It means putting a tube into the abdomen and then washing fluid in and out to keep the toxic substances in the blood down. It's not uncomfortable and you'll be taught to do it yourself for when you get home.

Patient: How long will I have to stay in hospital?

Doctor: You'll be in for about a week. With this method of dialysis you can walk about and live a reasonably normal life.

Patient: Shall I have to stop working, Doctor?

Doctor: Just remind me. What do you do?[15]

Patient: I'm a bus conductor.

Doctor: Well, I think it might prove difficult for you. I'd advise you to get a lighter job but we'll see how you get on.[16]

Patient: Shall I have to use this for the rest of my life?

Doctor: Well, there are changes and improvements in treatment all the time. We will take a specimen of your blood and put you on the computer for a kidney transplant. When a suitable kidney comes, we will do a kidney transplant operation. This will make life a lot easier and there are new drugs now to prevent the body rejecting the new kidney. So there are several ways of helping you. We'll just have to see how you get on.

Patient: Thank you Doctor.

Explanations

1. **water:** urine.
2. **keep getting up:** frequently get out of bed to urinate.
3. **been sick:** vomited.
4. **puffed up:** swollen.
5. **groggy:** unwell.
6. **a stone:** roughly 6.34 kg (see page xi).
7. **cleared up:** got better.
8. **not unpleasant:** In English when you have two negatives, known as a double negative, it creates a middle way, meaning not a positive, 'a pleasant diet', but not a negative, 'an unpleasant diet'. So here, 'not unpleasant' means a fairly acceptable diet.
9. **irreversible:** It is best to avoid phrases like this when speaking to most patients. Here the doctor quickly explains in more simple language what an irreversible condition means.
10. **I'm afraid:** These words signal to the patient regret. The phrase 'I'm afraid', is used to introduce news which is unwelcome, bad.
11. **keep an eye on you:** keep a frequent check on you.
12. **gather:** understand, believe.
13. **feeling dreadful:** an emotional phrase to express feeling very unwell.
14. **can't keep on like this:** can't continue in this condition.
15. **what do you do?:** what is your job?
16. **you get on:** you progress.

13. Man, aged 36

Follow-up in Cardiac Clinic. Junior doctor present with Consultant.

Doctor: Hello again, Mr Waites. We met last week, didn't we? I've been telling my colleague here about you. I've seen the results of the tests but there are just one or two points I'd like you to clarify for me and for the benefit of Dr Granger. You did say that this pain and discomfort has troubled you for nearly eight months and is getting worse?

Patient: That's right, Doctor. And since I saw you last week I had a really bad turn[1] after breakfast.

Doctor: Can I get you to describe the character of the pain – or in other words, tell us what it is like exactly?

Patient: It is not always a pain as such; often just a feeling of discomfort in the chest, like someone pressing on my chest.

Doctor: Does the discomfort go anywhere else?

Patient: Not really, although I do get a numbness in my leg with it.

Doctor: Last week you mentioned that it often came on when walking but not always. Can you remember what you are most commonly doing when it comes on?

Patient: I've been thinking about that since you asked me the last time I was here and usually it's after my evening meal and when I go to bed at night. I've also noticed it when I have sex with my wife. I very rarely get it at work.

Doctor: Well, it seems to me that perhaps the pain comes on as often when you are not exercising as when you are.

Patient: Yes, I'm sure that's true, Doctor.

Doctor: Could you just remind me what else you notice when you get this pain?

Patient: Like I told you last time, I do get palpitations[2] sometimes.

Doctor: By which you mean?

Patient: A strong banging in my chest as if my heart was going to come out.

Doctor: What about your breathing when you have the pain?

Patient: I don't notice any difference.

Doctor: Now what would happen if you and I went for a walk up the hill to the station?

Patient: What now?

Doctor: No, I just meant if we were to walk what do you think would happen? Could you keep up with[3] me if I walked fast?

Patient: Oh yes. Last summer I climbed Ben Nevis.[4]

Doctor: Mmm. Well, as I said, we've had the result of the tests and this discussion today has been very helpful. I'm happy to be able to reassure you about your heart which is essentially normal apart from one minor problem. One of the valves of your heart (and you've got four) leaks a little. This leaking produces an extra noise in the heart which we call a heart murmur. Although there is this murmur there, it doesn't interfere with the functioning of your heart and I'm quite sure it won't interfere with your enjoyment of life or length of life.

Patient: Is there anything you can do about it?

Doctor: Well, although we could give you medication for the palpitations, it isn't really necessary as they are not in the least bit dangerous. They're a nuisance but they may disappear of their own accord. So what I'm really saying is: this is a nuisance but only a nuisance. It's not dangerous and I want you to lead an entirely normal life. Do anything you want to do. The only one precaution is to tell any surgeon who wants to do an operation or dentist who wants to take out a tooth that you do need an antibiotic in order to prevent any infection getting on to the leaking valve.

Well now, Mr Waites. Is there anything you'd like to ask me?[5]

Patient: Do you think I've had this since birth?

Doctor: No, I don't think so but it is possible you were born with a tendency to develop this problem. Right, Mr Waites, I'll write to your doctor about all this. I don't think I need to see you on a regular basis as there's nothing seriously wrong but I'd be happy to see you again if your doctor would like you to.

Patient: Thank you Doctor. That's a relief.

Explanations

1. **a bad turn:** an attack of symptoms.
2. **palpitations:** this word is used by patients to mean different things so the doctor asks for clarification.
3. **keep up with:** walk as fast as.

4. **Ben Nevis:** the highest mountain in the UK.
5. This is a good question to ask patients to give them an opportunity of expressing fears, seeking clearer explanations, etc.

Letter to GP from Consultant

Cardiology Department
Royal Victoria Infirmary
Newcastle upon Tyne

7 December 1999

Dr Crisp
Abbotts Health Centre
14 Crispin Way
Newcastle upon Tyne

Dear Dr Crisp

R Waites (M) 4 6 63, 15 Faber Road, Newcastle upon Tyne

Thank you for asking me to see this man and for your helpful letter about him. He gives a history of chest discomfort which has been present for 8 months and is getting progressively worse. Although the chest discomfort usually occurs with exercise it can occur after eating and after sexual intercourse. The pain is sometimes associated with palpitations but he has not noticed any associated shortness of breath.

In the past he had pneumonia as a child and has also had an appendicectomy. I note that he smokes quite heavily and drinks a bottle of whisky per week. There is no family history of coronary artery disease.

On examination he is normotensive and there is no evidence

cont'd

of heart failure. His pulse is 80 regular and of normal character. His apex beat is normal on auscultation. He has normal heart sounds but has a late systolic murmur, maximal at the apex. It radiates to the left sternal edge. The remainder of the physical examination is normal and there are no stigmata of infective endocarditis or of liver disease. His investigations show a normal chest X-ray. His resting ECG shows some non-specific ST segment and T-wave changes in the inferior leads. It is otherwise normal. His echocardiogram shows a normal left ventricular cavity, normal aorta and left atrium. The pattern movement of the mitral valve suggests a prolapse of the valve. The left ventricular wall movements are quite normal.

I think it is likely that this man has a myxomatous degeneration of his mitral valve which is causing mitral regurgitation. This is of no haemodynamic importance and he should be encouraged to lead an entirely normal life. The only precaution he needs is for antibiotic cover for any potentially septic procedures.

Yours sincerely

Dr P Stevens MD FRCP
Consultant Physician & Cardiologist

14. Woman, aged 43

Presenting with a 3 cm lump in the upper, outer, quadrant of the left breast. She had noticed the lump 10 days previously and visited her GP who referred her to the local breast clinic.

Doctor: Your GP says you've been to see him about a lump[1] in your breast. So, when did you first notice this lump?

Patient: Ten days ago. I was lying in the bath examining my breasts and I was shocked to find this lump...

Doctor: Have you been examining your breasts for a long time?

Patient: Well, for a good few years but more since my mother ...

she died six months ago of breast cancer and I've been scared[2] of getting it.

Doctor: How old was she?

Patient: Sixty-five.

Doctor: Are you married?

Patient: Yes, but we split up[3] nine months ago. He went off with another woman and I'm on my own looking after my two children.

Doctor: How old are they?

Patient: A girl 14 and a boy 12.

Doctor: Have you ever had any serious illnesses or operations?

Patient: No. I've been lucky.

Doctor: Are you taking any medication, any tablets of any kind?

Patient: No. I try to avoid them if possible.

Doctor: Well, I'd like to examine you so if you could please take off your clothes above the waist and lie on the couch. I'll be with you in a minute.

On examination, a non-tender 3 cm discrete lump in the upper, outer, quadrant of the left breast was found. No nodes were palpable in the axillae or supraclavicular fossae. On needle aspiration it proved to be a solid lump. Glass slides prepared for cytological examination.

After examination:

Doctor: I suspect this may be a tumour of the breast.

Patient: Do you mean breast cancer doctor?

Doctor: Yes, but I cannot be absolutely sure until the results of the cytology and mammography are available.

Patient: But if it is, shall I lose my breast? I dread[4] that...

Doctor: No, I think that is very unlikely. It seems to be quite a small cancer so we should be able to avoid a mastectomy and treat it by local excision followed by a course of radiotherapy if it, in fact, proves to be a breast cancer on the tests.

Patient: I don't care what it is so long as I don't lose my breast. Will I need chemotherapy?

Doctor: That depends on the results from the operation. If the lymph

> nodes in the armpit have tumour in them then we usually suggest chemotherapy but it will depend very much on how you feel about chemotherapy.

Patient: My mother had chemotherapy and she lost all her hair.

Doctor: Yes, that can happen with some types of chemotherapy, but it depends on the drugs which are used. The drugs we use now in the treatment of breast cancer rarely cause hair loss.

Patient: Shall I be able to keep on[5] working while I'm having the treatment? You see I need the money with two young children.

Doctor: Most people are able to carry on[6] working whilst they are having treatment, but you will need to take about two weeks off for the operation. Anyway at the moment I am not even sure that this is a breast cancer. Could you bring a friend with you when I see you in the next clinic? It is always helpful to have somebody else listening so that you can compare notes afterwards.

Patient: Yes, I'll bring my friend next time. Thank you very much doctor and see you in five days' time.

Follow-up Clinic:

Doctor: Hello Mrs Baxter, how are you today?

Patient: Dreading the news doctor.

Doctor: Well, the results of all the tests show that the lump is a breast cancer so we shall now have to talk about the best way of dealing with it. I know you don't like the thought of losing your breast so I think we should do a local excision of the breast cancer and avoid a mastectomy.

Patient: Is it safe? Is it as safe as having a mastectomy?

Doctor: Yes it is, if you follow it with a course of radiotherapy.

Patient: Its not just me. I've got the children to think about. Shall I live as long if I don't have a mastectomy?

Doctor: Yes, the survival prospects are identical for a mastectomy and local excision. So is that what you would like? Local excision of the lump under general anaesthetic followed by a course of radiotherapy?

Patient: Yes doctor. Will you do it?

Doctor: Yes. I'll arrange for you to come in next week, next Tuesday and we shall do the operation on Wednesday. You will be assessed by the anaesthetists before the operation and the breast cancer nurse will see you now to answer any questions that you may have.

Patient: Thank you.

The lump is excised from the breast and the axillary nodes are cleared. The drains are removed three days after the operation and the patient is discharged.

Follow-up Clinic (Mrs Baxter comes with her sister):

Doctor: Hello Mrs Baxter. Well, how've you been since I last saw you?

Patient: Well, a bit low and my armpit is rather sore. What did you find at the operation?

Doctor: Well, we removed the tumour. It was a 1.3 cm diameter ductal carcinoma, grade 1, and two out of seventeen lymph nodes that were removed from the armpit contain some tumour.

Patient: Does that mean that it has spread to the rest of my body?

Doctor: No, not at all. This was a small breast cancer of only 1.3 cm and it is a very good grade. However, two of the lymph nodes had tumour in them, so that does raise the possibility that there may be microscopic deposits of tumour elsewhere in the body and therefore it would be safer if you had some type of drug therapy.

Patient: You mentioned radiotherapy before. Do I still need that?

Doctor: Yes, you will need radiotherapy. That will reduce the risk of any recurrence in the breast but radiotherapy has very few side-effects. It is the drug therapy that is probably more important to consider at this stage, as I mentioned to you before, because the lymph nodes have some tumour in them. It is possible, although by no means certain, that there may be tumour cells elsewhere in the body.

Mrs Baxter's Sister: Do you mean she will have radiotherapy as well as chemotherapy?

Doctor: Yes. We usually give chemotherapy for about six months and then give a course of radiotherapy after it is finished. The chemotherapy is given once a month and in most cases tends to make you feel sick and unwell for about three days, so that means that you will feel unwell for about three or four days a month. The side-effects vary considerably from one person to another.

Patient: Shall I need to stay in hospital for the chemotherapy?

Doctor: No. You will have a blood test before each treatment. The chemotherapy is given through a drip in your arm, so you will be here for about two hours each time. Then after the sixth course of chemotherapy has been given we shall need to start the radiotherapy.

Patient: Do you think I shall be able to carry on working during this time?

Mrs Baxter's Sister: You know she has two young children.

Doctor: Yes, you should be able to work during the period. If the chemotherapy is given on a Friday then the patients that I know tend to go back to work on the Tuesday.

Patient: Will I need any other treatment doctor?

Doctor: It may be worth considering giving you tamoxifen as well as the chemotherapy. At the moment we are not sure whether this additional treatment is of any benefit so we are asking patients whether they wish to go into a trial so that we can find out whether tamoxifen or other hormone drugs should be added to chemotherapy. You do not need to make a decision about this at the moment but I will ask the Oncologist to discuss this with you when you see her.

Patient: Do you think I've got a chance[7] doctor? I just want to be sure about the children.

Doctor: The trouble with breast cancer is that it is unpredictable, but you had a small cancer with a good grade and only two nodes were involved. I think you really do have a very good outlook.

Patient: Am I going to die?

Doctor: No.

Patient: Well, I'm going to fight this.

Doctor: That's the best way. You seem a strong person.

Patient: Oh yes, I've always been fit and I have so much to live for.

Doctor: Good, well I'll see you next week and I will introduce you to the Oncology team. Good luck.

Explanations

1. **lump:** mass, tumour.
2. **scared:** frightened.
3. **split up:** separated.
4. **dread:** fear.
5. **keep on:** continue.
6. **carry on:** continue.
7. **a chance:** any hope of surviving.

15. Man, aged 73

Man complained of alternating constipation and diarrhoea with bloodstained stools and loss of weight. Examination showed a mobile mass on the left iliac fossa. Barium enema shows cancer of the pelvic colon.

Doctor: Well, Mr Longwood, you've been having trouble with your bowels for a long time. The last time you came to hospital, we did an X-ray and this showed that there is a growth[1] which is causing the bleeding.

Patient: Is it serious, Doctor?

Doctor: It will be if we leave it, so I would recommend you to have an operation to remove the growth. You will be in hospital for about two to three weeks and then we'll see you for regular check-ups.

Patient: Aren't I too old to have an operation?

Doctor: Oh no. Age is no bar[2] to surgery these days. We consider each patient individually. Some patients are young at ninety and others are old at sixty.

Patient: I won't have to have a bag,[3] will I?[4]

Doctor: Fortunately not. After the operation you should have no trouble with your bowels.

Patient: Shall I need any other kind of treatment?

Doctor: No. The operation should clear up[5] the trouble. So I'll write to your doctor and tell him we are bringing you into hospital to have an operation. I shall probably see you in the ward in about ten days' time.

Patient: Thank you, Doctor.

Explanations

1. **a growth:** a mass, cancer.
2. **age is no bar:** age is no obstacle; here the success of surgery does not depend on age.
3. **to have a bag:** a bag to empty the bowel following a colostomy.
4. **I won't ... a bag, will I?:** Note this form of negative statement followed by a positive question tag. The patient hopes for a negative answer. He is seeking reassurance.
5. **clear up:** remedy.

Letter to GP from Consultant

Geriatric Department
Whittington Hospital
London N19

4 April 2001

Dr C Young
6 Melburn Grove
N19

Dear Dr Young

Charles Longwood (M) 1/2/1928, 24 Highgate Avenue, N19

The barium enema on this patient confirmed the presence of a stenosing Ca of the pelvic colon. I have discussed him with

(cont'd)

> Mr Sanderson and he will admit him in the next few days for surgery. I've told Mr Longwood that he has a growth and needs surgery and that we should be quite optimistic about the future. I have assured him that he will not need a colostomy.
>
> Yours sincerely
>
> Paul Newton
> Consultant Geriatrician

16. Man, aged 56

Long-term cigarette smoker, diagnosed with lung cancer 6 months ago, now referred by the chest physicians complaining of low back pain. He comes to the clinic at the hospice[1] for the first time with his wife.

Doctor: Good morning Mr Malin, I'm Dr Smith. Would you like to take a seat here, and your wife can have this one. I understand you saw Dr Lamb, the chest consultant, in the clinic with Sandra, one of the nurses who works with me. They thought perhaps I might be able to help you with this back pain you've been having.

Patient: Yes, I've had the pain for six weeks now and it's getting worse. My GP gave me some arthritis tablets. They helped at first, but now they seem to have worn off[2] and the pain is stopping me from sleeping. He took some X-rays at the beginning and said they looked OK.

Doctor: Have you got pain anywhere else apart from the low back?

Patient: No. Everything else seems OK.

Doctor: And the actual back pain, it's there all the time?

Patient: Yes, virtually[3] all the time.

Doctor: Have you had any weakness in your legs, or any odd sensations like pins and needles?

Patient: No, nothing like that.

Doctor: And you are opening your bowels and passing water without any problems? What I mean is do you know when you want to go?

Patient: Yes, all of that is just the same as usual.

Doctor: Otherwise any other problems? Breathing's OK? Eating alright?

Patient: Yes, my breathing has been a lot better since they gave me the X-ray treatment at the hospital a few months ago.

Doctor: Are you taking any medicines apart from the Voltarol your GP gave you?

Patient: No.

Doctor: And apart from this recent problem with your lungs, no other serious illnesses in the past?

Patient: No, I've always been as fit as a fiddle.[4] That's why I couldn't believe it at first when I became ill. I suppose it's all down[5] to the smoking.

Doctor: Well, let's have a look at you. Can you get undressed, just leave your underpants on. Would you like your wife to stay while I examine you?

Patient: She's seen it all before. (*Patient and his wife laugh.*)

After examining the patient, when the patient is fully dressed again.

Doctor: Do sit down. Now let me explain what I think is going on. You are certainly very tender over the bones in your lower back. There's no sign of any problems in the legs. It seems that the problem is coming from the bones in the lower back.

Patient: Is it something to do with the lung cancer I had earlier this year? I know it can spread.

Doctor: Wel, I suspect it might be but we need to do some tests first to find out. Although the X-rays were normal, that is not the most sensitive test for this sort of problem. What we need is a bone scan. It's a very simple test. They give you a small injection in your arm and a few hours later they scan you with a machine a little bit like an X-ray machine. It doesn't hurt. The scan shows any areas of bone that are abnormal. If it shows an abnormality in your low back then we can arrange for the radiotherapy doctors to see you again and give you treatment just like they did with your lung.

Patient's wife: Then it is quite serious now.

Doctor: Well, as I am sure the doctors at the time told you both, we cannot cure this disease. What we aim to do is to control any symptoms it might cause you.

Patient's wife: Yes I know – they did say that, and Dr Lamb said the same in the clinic. He told us that you are a specialist in controlling symptoms.

Doctor: Now while we wait for the scan, you need a better pain killer to keep you comfortable. What I would suggest is a low dose of morphine. It is a very safe but strong painkiller. The only side-effect we need to worry about is constipation. You will have to take a laxative to counteract this. Keep on taking the arthritis drug, Voltarol, that your GP gave you. The two drugs together often work better than either alone.

Patient: Doctor I know this might sound silly but I won't get addicted to it, will I?

Doctor: Absolutely not. Thousands of patients just like you take morphine for pain, and there is no evidence whatsoever that they become addicted. And if the scan is positive and you have radiotherapy then you will probably stop the morphine after a few weeks, once the radiotherapy has taken effect. I'll see you in clinic with the results of the scan. Have you any other questions or worries before you go?

Patient: No, I think I understand.

Doctor: Well, it's been very nice meeting you, and I hope you'll feel a lot better on the new painkiller. Sandra will keep in touch with you at home and if you have any problems before your appointment just let her know.

Follow-up clinic:

Doctor: Hello. Take a seat. How have you been?

Patient: Well, the pain has gone and I've had no problems with my bowels. The laxative seems to work.

Patient's wife: Yes, it's wonderful – he's a different man.

Doctor: Good. The result of the scan is as I thought it would be. There is an abnormal area in the lower back.

Patient: So the cancer has spread there?

Doctor: Yes it has, and I am sure that some radiotherapy will get the pain well under control and then you won't need to take the medicines. I have arranged for you to see the radiotherapist this Monday and he says he will treat you the same day. You've been treated before so you know what it is like. There shouldn't be any real problems.

Patient: Thank you doctor. It's a relief to know its going to be sorted out.

Doctor: That's no problem. I won't make a formal follow-up appointment. Your nurse, Sandra, will keep in touch with you at home and if there are any further problems she or your GP will let me know and I can see you again, either here or at home if necessary. She will let me know how you get on after your radiotherapy and she'll be able to give you advice on tailing off[6] your painkillers.

Patient: Yes she's wonderful; it just makes us feel safe knowing she's around.

Doctor: Goodbye then, and good luck on Monday.

Explanations

1. **hospice:** a home for the care of the terminally ill
2. **worn off:** be less effective
3. **virtually:** almost
4. **as fit as a fiddle:** in very good health
5. **all down to:** as a result of
6. **tailing off:** reducing the amount

17. Woman, aged 29

Doctor: I see from your notes you were in hospital 10 years ago with thyroid trouble.[1]

Patient: Yes, that's right. And now I've got stomach trouble and my doctor sent me here.

Doctor: What has actually been happening since the thyroid trouble?

Patient: All sorts of things. I've been feeling very depressed for a year.

Doctor: Did you go to your doctor?

Patient: Yes, when it got bad. He gave me some Valium tablets to slow me down but they slowed me to a halt.[2] I didn't do anything but sleep.

Doctor: Did they affect you in any other way?

Patient: Yes, I got indigestion.

Doctor: Did he give you anything for that?

Patient: Yes, he gave me some medicine and then it was all right.

Doctor: How does the indigestion affect you?

Patient: All the food stays up here (indicating chest).

Doctor: When do you get it?

Patient: Two to three hours after food.

Doctor: What is it like? A pain?

Patient: Yes, a pain.

Doctor: What kind? Burning, stabbing?[3]

Patient: It feels like some wind there and I want to get rid of it.[4]

Doctor: Do you belch?[5]

Patient: Not much.

Doctor: Does it bother you at night?[6]

Patient: No.

Doctor: It comes on when you are hungry?[7]

Patient: Yes, I have a terrible pain in my stomach and I feel I'll collapse if I don't eat straight away.[8]

Doctor: How is your appetite?

Patient: Very poor.

Doctor: Did you always have a bad one?

Patient: No, it started to deteriorate ten years ago.[9]

Doctor: Has it changed much in the last few months?

Patient: I think the medicine must push the food down and then I feel hungry.

Doctor: What about your weight?

Patient: I'm losing weight.

Doctor: How much do you weigh now?

Patient: Eight stone, one pound.[10]

Doctor: And how much did you weigh a year ago?

Patient: Nine stone.[11]

Doctor: What about your bowels?

Patient: Terrible.[12]

Doctor: In what way?

Patient: I'm constipated.

Doctor: How often do you have them opened?

Patient: Only when I take medicine.[13]

Doctor: Every day?

Patient: No, every other day.

Doctor: Does warm weather affect you?

Patient: No, I prefer warm weather but it makes me sweat.

Doctor: Do you always sweat?

Patient: Yes, but more recently. ·

Doctor: All over your body?

Patient: Yes, all over.

Doctor: Do you feel depressed, nervous, edgy,[14] irritable?

Patient: I was worse before I got my job.

Doctor: When did you start that?

Patient: A month ago.

Doctor: Have you been fidgety,[15] have your hands been shaky?

Patient: When I was coming here.

Doctor: At times of stress?

Patient: Yes. And when something riles[16] me.

Doctor: Any trouble with your eyes?

Patient: No.

Doctor: Periods[17] regular?

Patient: Every month since I had my baby.

Doctor: When was that?

Patient: Five years ago.

Doctor: Do you feel restless?

Patient: I couldn't concentrate till I got my job but now I have to.

Doctor: Is there anything else you've noticed?

Patient: No.

Doctor: Has anyone in your family had thyroid trouble?

Patient: No. I have one sister and two brothers.

Doctor: Are they well?

Patient: Yes.

Clinical notes

- Woman 29 years
- Overactive thyroid 10 years ago
- Stomach trouble
- Depressed 1 yr Valium. Sleepy
- Dyspepsia 2/3 hrs after food.
- *Appetite*   Poor
- *Wt* 1998   9 st 0 lb[18]
      1999   8 st 1 lb[19]
- *Bowels*   Constipated
- *Periods*   Regular   1 son (5)
- *Family*   1S + 2B   A & W
            Parents   A & W

O/E

- Rather staring eyes
- EOM full
- No lid lag or retraction
- Thyroid palpable
- ® lobe enlarged 3 × 4 cm
- No bruit
- No tremor
- Warm dry hands
- CVS   P   72 reg
         Ht   not enlarged
         Ht sounds   √
         BP $\dfrac{120}{80}$
- RS   √
- AS   √

| – CNS | Reflexes not exaggerated |
| | Plantar ↓ ↓ |

Investigations
- TSH
- Hb
- WBC
- ESR
- Ba meal
- CXR
- Neck XR
- Δ? Peptic ulcer
- ? Thyrotoxicosis
- ? Anxiety state.

Explanations

1. **trouble:** This word is widely used. Here it means 'disturbance'. A doctor often begins speaking to a patient with the words, 'What's the trouble?', i.e. what is worrying you? What is wrong with you?

2. **slow me down:** calm me down. **slowed me to a halt:** slowed me down to a complete stop.

3. **what kind:** Although the patient has admitted she has a pain, the doctor has to suggest different *kinds* of pain. See pages 175–177 for the language of pain.

4. **wind:** flatulence. **to get rid of:** lose

5. **belch:** bring up wind.

6. **bother:** give you trouble, upset.

7. **It comes on when you are hungry?:** Notice this form of question. It is really a statement but in speech the rising intonation at the end shows that the speaker wishes to have confirmation of his statement so it *is* a kind of question.

8. **straight away:** immediately, at once.

9. **deteriorate:** get worse.

10. **eight stone, one pound:** See page xi.

11. **nine stone:** The patient has lost thirteen pounds in weight, which is a lot.
12. **terrible:** very bad.
13. **medicine:** laxative, aperient.
14. **edgy:** nervous, irritable.
15. **fidgety:** nervously touching and playing with things.
16. **riles:** annoys, makes me angry.
17. **periods:** menstruation.
18. **9 st 0 lb:** nine stone.
19. **8 st 1 lb:** eight stone and one pound.

18. Woman, aged 52

Doctor: You come from Cyprus?
Patient: Yes, but I've been in England for twenty-three years.
Doctor: Are you married to an Englishman?
Patient: I was, but we were divorced fifteen years ago.
Doctor: Well. Tell me about your trouble.
Patient: Two hours after eating I get pain and when I bend I get it.
Doctor: Do you bring up liquid?
Patient: No.
Doctor: Do you have the taste of sour liquid in your mouth?
Patient: Yes, terrible.
Doctor: Do you ever vomit?
Patient: Not really.
Doctor: Do you belch?
Patient: A little.
Doctor: Do you have this pain every day?
Patient: No.
Doctor: Does it wake you up at night?
Patient: No.
Doctor: If you drink something hot, does it affect you?
Patient: I feel it burning as it goes down.
Doctor: Do you feel acid as well as burning?
Patient: No.
Doctor: Have you anything else that worries you?

Patient: No.

Doctor: What about your weight?

Patient: I've put on weight – four pounds.[1]

Doctor: How's your appetite?

Patient: Very good.

Doctor: Does any particular food upset you?

Patient: Yes. I was fasting[2] for three days for my religion and then I went to my sister's and had some fish and chips.

Doctor: Had you ever been upset by fried things before?

Patient: No.

Doctor: Do you regularly fast?

Patient: Twice a year for my religion.

Doctor: Have you had similar trouble before?

Patient: Never.

Doctor: Have you any children?

Patient: No.

Doctor: How are the bowels?

Patient: Irregular.

Doctor: Have you ever passed blood?

Patient: No.

Doctor: How's the water?

Patient: Normal.

Doctor: Do you ever get up at night to pass water?

Patient: No.

Doctor: Do you still see your periods?

Patient: No, they finished two years ago.

Doctor: Did you ever have a discharge or bleeding between your periods?

Patient: No.

Doctor: Do you smoke?

Patient: No.

Doctor: Drink?

Patient: Occasionally.

Doctor: Any serious illnesses?

Patient: I had an ectopic pregnancy fifteen years ago.

Doctor: Has anyone in your family stomach trouble?

Patient: No, but my mother had gallstones and had an operation here and my sister and my brother have gallstones.

Doctor: What about your father?

Patient: He died when I was six but I don't know why.

Doctor: Do you work?

Patient: I'm a dressmaker but I haven't worked for a year. I'm having a rest.

Doctor: Do you live alone?

Patient: Yes.

Doctor: How can you manage to live without working?

Patient: I have a tenant.[3]

Doctor: Do you worry about things?

Patient: No. I used to worry but not now. I know it's not worth it.

Doctor: I'd like to examine you. It sounds as though this is not gallstone but stomach trouble.

The doctor gave the following instructions during the clinical examination:

- Take a deep breath in and out (measures chest expansion).
- Breathe through your mouth (listens to breath sounds).
- I'm going to shake your stomach (listens for splash).
- Let me look at your ankles. Are they ever swollen? (looks for oedema).
- Bend your knees (elicits knee jerks).
- I'm going to tickle your feet (elicits plantar response).
- I'm going to take some blood. You'll feel a jab.
- I can't find anything seriously wrong with you. I think this is due to the weakness of the muscle at the lower end of your gullet[4] which is allowing acid to come back into your gullet. We'd better do an X-ray of the stomach and gallbladder as you have this tendency in your family. We'll check on the blood as well. Avoid bending. The stomach should not be empty of food for too long. Try to eat little and often. I'll give you some medicine to take after meals and some tablets to take before meals. I'll see you in three weeks when I've got the results of the X-rays and tests.

Clinical notes

O/E
- CVS   P 80

              Ht not enlarged

              Ht sounds

              BP $\dfrac{130}{90}$

- RS   NAD
- Abd   Slight epigastric tenderness

              Succussion splash
- CNS   NAD

              No enlarged lymph nodes
- Breasts normal

Investigations
- Hb
- WBC
- ESR
- CXR
- Barium meal
- Ultrasound gallbladder
- Δ?   Gastro-oesophageal reflux from hiatus hernia
- □??   Gallstones

Treatment
Advice + Mucaine p.c., Maxolon a.c.

Explanations
1. **four pounds:** See page xi.
2. **fasting:** going without food.
3. **a tenant:** a person who pays rent for a room.
4. **gullet:** oesophagus.

Letter to GP from Consultant

Whittington Hospital
Highgate Hill
London N19

15 February 2000

Dr Peter Owen
6 Kentish Town Road
London NW5

Dear Dr Owen

Elena Cooper (F) 4 7 48, 3 Downside Terrace, NW5

Thank you for your letter about this patient. For the past five weeks she has noticed regurgitation, heartburn and belching coming on two hours after food or on bending. Hot tea burns her. She is gaining weight. Her symptoms seem to have been precipitated by a three day religious fast terminated by fish and chips! She has had milder similar symptoms in the past after large meals. There is a strong family history of gallstones in her mother, sister and brother.

On examination there were no significant abnormalities. I think this is gastro-oesophageal reflux with a possible hiatus hernia. I have ordered a barium meal and an abdominal ultrasound. I have meanwhile given her a supply of Maxolon and Mucaine until I next see her and have advised her about her eating habits.

Yours sincerely

David Layton
Consultant Physician

19. Woman, aged 44

Patient had visited her GP 24 hours earlier complaining of weakness. He refers her to hospital.

Doctor: Good morning Mrs Baxter. I'm Dr Crosland. Your GP asked me to see you at short notice because the blood test he did was abnormal. Did he explain this to you?

Patient: I didn't really understand what he was saying. I'm very frightened because he told me to come here so quickly it must be serious.

Doctor: Yes, well we're not yet certain about the diagnosis but the blood test did show that you were very anaemic and there seem to be some abnormal white blood cells. We'll need to do some more tests and I'll explain about them later. May I ask you some questions?

Patient: Yes.

Doctor: Can I start at the beginning? Can I check your age?

Patient: Forty-four.

Doctor: What sort of work do you do?

Patient: I'm a teacher.

Doctor: So I can assume you haven't been exposed to any nasty toxic chemicals?

Patient: Well, we get the fumes from the photocopier but nothing else.

Doctor: Well now, tell me how long you've been unwell.

Patient: Really only about two weeks.

Doctor: What were the main problems?

Patient: I just got weaker and weaker. I ran out of energy and fainted in the doctor's surgery yesterday.

Doctor: Have you had any bruising?

Patient: Yes, I noticed some on my thighs and one on my forearm where I had my blood taken.

Doctor: Oh dear. Any bleeding from the gums?

Patient: No.

Doctor: Have you had any problem with infections recently?

Patient: No—well, I had 'flu about two months ago.

Doctor: Has anyone in your family had blood problems?

Patient: No.

Patient's sister: Oh, didn't granny[1] have anaemia and was treated with iron?

Doctor: Mmm. I was thinking of more serious blood diseases.

Patient: Not that we know of.

Doctor: Have you had any serious illnesses in the past?

Patient: No.

Doctor: Are there any other things you think I should know about?

Patient: No.

Doctor: May I examine you?

Doctor examines patient.

Clinical Notes

— Woman 44

— Pallor but no jaundice

— Bruises on forearm at site of venepuncture. Several on thighs. One on buttock and shoulder

— Gums healthy

— No enlarged lymph nodes

— P 94 reg

— BP $\dfrac{110}{75}$

— soft systolic ejection murmur LSE? flow murmur

— C. clear

— No ankle oedema

— Abd. No hepatomegaly

— Spleen palpable 2 cm below costal margin

The patient is told to dress.

Patient: Do you think it is leukaemia, doctor?

Doctor: Well, I've still got to take more blood to confirm the diagnosis but I've seen the results of the previous test and I'm afraid there is a 95% chance that it is leukaemia. Have you any questions before we take the extra blood?

Patient's sister: Can she have a bone marrow transplant?

Doctor: First of all we have to be 100% sure of the diagnosis. Then I will explain to you all the possible treatment options. We need to find you a bed straight away. You're very anaemic and we will give you a blood transfusion with your permission. I'd also like to do a bone marrow test.

Patient: What's that? Where would it be taken from?

Doctor: Normally from this bone. (indicating the posterior iliac crest).

Patient: Will I have an anaesthetic?

Doctor: A local anaesthetic. We suck out a little of the marrow. When we do this it produces a very strange pain which lasts only seconds, but it is important you know what it is.

Patient's sister: Are there any complications to the bone marrow test?

Doctor: No, remarkably few. It may bleed and very rarely you can get an infection.

Patient: All right. Can we get on with it?[2]

Next day in a quiet room at the hospital:

Doctor: I want to talk to you and your husband here privately. We got back the cell marker studies from a special centre and I'm afraid that these and the bone marrow test do confirm that you have a leukaemia.

Patient: I see.

Patient's husband: Can this be treated?

Doctor: Yes. There are several forms of treatment. It is important that you understand the type of leukaemia you have. It is acute myeloid leukaemia.

Patient: Can it be cured?

Doctor: I can't promise you a cure but there is real hope.

Patient: Will I have to have chemotherapy?

Doctor: Yes, we would offer you a form of chemotherapy.

Patient: Will I go bald?

Doctor: Yes, I'm afraid that will happen with the aggressive chemotherapy we use.

Patient: Will my hair grow again?

Doctor: Yes, once you've finished the treatment. May I tell you about the different forms of treatment?

Patient: All right.

Doctor: This type of leukaemia can be treated in a number of ways and we ask all patients whether they would be prepared to take part in MRC[3] trials. I have some written information here that I'd like to go through[4] with you.

Patient studies information.

Patient: This all looks very complicated.

Doctor: Yes, it does but I can explain all the abbreviations to make it clearer. The basic idea is that we need to give you large doses of chemotherapy for several weeks. The exact pattern depends on which part of the trial you go into.

Patient: Can I have treatment without going into trials?

Doctor: Yes, of course, and you would be given the best possible treatment.

Patient: What's this about a Hickman Line?

Doctor: It is a special sort of drip we use. It is put into the chest wall and runs up under the skin and back into a vein in the neck and back just above the heart. A surgeon does it and it is more comfortable than having many drips in your hands and arms. Well, this has been a shock for you and your husband and I know you need to support each other. I will ask nurse to bring you some tea and I suggest you stay here quietly and think about it all. The nurses are nearby and we do have a psychologist to help you if you need one. I shall come back later to see you both.

Explanations

1. **granny:** grandmother.
2. **get on with it:** do the test soon.
3. **MRC:** Medical Research Council.
4. **go through:** explain.

20. Woman, aged 18

Referred by GP, complaining of rash all over body.

Doctor: **What can I do for you?**

Patient: I have got a nasty[1] rash all over.

Doctor: **When did it start?**

Patient: Well, I have always had flaky skin on my elbows and knees for as long as I can remember. Sometimes I get scaly scalp too, with lots of dandruff. But this rash started about four weeks ago. Suddenly, I noticed lots of little red spots all over my tummy and back and they spread down my arms and legs and I have even got some on my face.

Doctor: **Are they itchy?[2]**

Patient: No, they just look terrible.

Doctor: **Have you ever seen anybody about the rash that you get on your elbows and knees?**

Patient: Yes, I went to my GP and he said it was psoriasis and gave me some cream to put on it, which normally helps. But this rash is different. I have never had anything like this before.

Doctor: **Before your rash came out did you have a sore throat?**

Patient: Yes, I had tonsillitis about six weeks ago and my GP gave me penicillin for it, and that cleared it up.[3] Do you think the sore throat has got anything to do with the rash?

Doctor: **Yes, sometimes the bacteria that cause a sore throat can make your psoriasis flare up.[4]**

Patient: Is this rash all over me the same as the psoriasis that I get on my elbows?

Doctor: **Yes, it is a form of psoriasis. Does anybody else in your family have psoriasis?**

Patient: My father has psoriasis and his father has psoriasis. My dad's psoriasis is bad because he has also got arthritis with it.

Doctor: **Do you get any joint problems?**

Patient: No, my joints are fine but I do have problems with my fingernails. Look.

Doctor: Have you ever been seriously ill in the past?

Patient: No.

Doctor: Are you on any medication at the moment?

Patient: No, except for these tablets that my GP said are antihistamines. He thought they would help with the rash.

Doctor: Are you putting any creams on the rash at the moment?

Patient: No, my usual psoriasis cream has run out.[5]

Doctor: What do you do for a living?

Patient: I am a secretary.

Doctor: Do you smoke?

Patient: About a packet a day.

Doctor: How much alcohol do you drink a day?

Patient: Oh, that depends; not much during the week. Occasionally I have a glass of wine at weekends, and sometimes I go out to the pub once a week.

Doctor: I need to have a look at your skin. Can you pop[6] next door, slip everything off except your bra and pants and pop yourself up on the bed please?

Doctor examines patient and finds widespread guttate psoriasis with some chronic plaque psoriasis on the elbows and knees.

Doctor: This is a flare up of your psoriasis which I suspect is being triggered by[7] your tonsillitis. Don't worry, we can get you better. I would like to do a throat swab and a blood test to see if that is the case. What you need is to have some light treatment to make your rash settle down.[8] You will have to come up to the hospital twice a week to the physiotherapy department to have UVB light. The department is open from about eight o'clock in the morning till about six o'clock at night. Do you think you could fit that in with your work?

Patient: Are you arranging for me to have sunbed treatment doctor?

Doctor: Yes, it is a form of sunbed treatment but the sunbeds we have in hospital are special and emit only UVB light. You will get a suntan though.

Patient: That sounds great; as long as it clears up[9] my rash I don't mind. When can I start?

Doctor: There is a slight wait, so I will give you this cream to be getting on with.[10] If you put it on twice a day to the areas where you've got the psoriasis, that will help. Take this form downstairs to the physiotherapy department and they will book you in for six weeks of UVB treatment. All the best.

Patient: Thank you very much doctor. Bye.

Explanations

1. **nasty:** unpleasant.
2. **itchy:** pruritus.
3. **cleared it up:** was effective.
4. **flare up:** suddenly become active.
5. **run out:** come to an end.
6. **pop:** colloquial expression meaning 'go next door' and 'get up on the bed'.
7. **triggered by:** precipitated by.
8. **settle down:** become quiescent.
9. **clears up:** removes.
10. **to be getting on with:** to use before the light treatment starts.

21. Woman, aged 22

Referred to the Rheumatology outpatient clinic, complaining of pain in her joints.

Doctor: Hello, I'm Dr Brown. I'm a Specialist Registrar in Rheumatology. Do come in and have a seat. How old are you now?

Patient: Twenty-two.

Doctor: And are you working?

Patient: No.

Doctor: You have been referred by your GP with joint pain. How long have you had this?

Patient: A long time.

Doctor: How many months would you say?

Patient: About six.

Doctor: And which joints have been a problem?

Patient: Virtually all of them.

Doctor: Is the pain worse at one time of the day?

Patient: Usually when I get up, while getting my kid ready.[1]

Doctor: And how long does the pain continue for?

Patient: About lunchtime.'

Doctor: Do the joints feel stiff?

Patient: Yeah,[2] really stiff first thing.[3]

Doctor: Have the joints ever been swollen?

Patient: No.

Doctor: When you went to see your GP about the joint pains, did she give you any medicines to try?

Patient: Yes. Some red tablets.

Doctor: Can you remember their name?

Patient: Burufen, or something, I think.

Doctor: Was it Brufen?

Patient: That's it.

Doctor: And did they help?

Patient: Not really.

Doctor: I'm going to ask you some general questions now. Please don't be surprised if they don't seem connected. How do you feel in yourself? Do you feel well?

Patient: No. I've been feeling knackered[4] for months.

Doctor: Have you been off your food[5] at all?

Patient: No, but I have lost half a stone.[6]

Doctor: Have you had any rashes?

Patient: Yeah. When I went to Spain my face came up all red and blotchy.[7] I thought it might have been the sun tan lotion, but it stayed like that for ages.[8]

Doctor: Whereabouts on the face was the rash?

Patient: Here, on my face and nose.

Doctor: Have you had excessive mouth ulcers recently?

Patient: Yeah, loads.[9]

Doctor: Any hair loss, I mean more than normal?

Patient: No.

Doctor: Do you find if you go out into the cold that your fingers change colour and become painful?

Patient: Yes. They have done for a few years.

Doctor: What colour do they go?

Patient: Sort of purple, and sometimes white, then red when I get back indoors.

Doctor: Do you ever experience excessively dry or gritty eyes or a dry mouth?

Patient: Only if I've left my contacts[10] in for too long.

Doctor: Have you had any fevers recently?

Patient: No.

Doctor: Do you get headaches?

Patient: No.

Doctor: Any problems with chest pain?

Patient: No.

Doctor: Have you had any illnesses or operations in the past?

Patient: Just my tonsils out.

Doctor: Have you had any problems with clots in the legs or on the lungs, or miscarriages?[11]

Patient: No.

Doctor: And how about your family? Do any diseases run in the family, for example, joint problems or lupus?

Patient: I think my Gran[12] had some sort of arthritis, affecting her knees, and had an operation, but nothing else.

Doctor: Do you live with anyone or on your own?

Patient: I live with my boyfriend.

Doctor: How many children do you have?

Patient: Just one.

Doctor: Do you drink any alcohol?

Patient: Only at weekends.

Doctor: How much do you usually have?

Patient: Just a few drinks on a Friday or Saturday.

Doctor: Do you smoke?

Patient: Yes.

Doctor: How many a day?

Patient: Fifteen to twenty.

Doctor: Are you taking any medicines at the moment?

Patient: No.

Doctor: We've covered most things, but have you had any other problems with your health recently, for example, problems with your breathing, cough, bowels, waterworks[13] or periods?[14]

Patient: No.

Doctor: Could I ask you now to slip your clothes off down to your underwear behind the curtain and climb up on the couch there. There's a blanket to keep you warm.

Dr Brown examined the patient's cardiovascular and respiratory systems, abdomen, joints and skin and did not detect any abnormality. The doctor explained to the patient the likely general nature of her joint problem but said that she would need to await further tests before being able to definitely confirm its precise nature. She asked her to provide a sample of urine and have blood taken for further tests and arranged to see the patient again in 4 weeks' time. The results of the investigations performed are shown below.

Clinical Notes

- Urinalysis: normal
- Hb $\quad$ 11.3×10^9/l $\quad$ MCV 90 fl
- WCC $\quad$ 7.8×10^9/l $\quad$ with lymphopenia
- Platelets $\quad$ 250×10^9/l
- ESR $\quad$ 78 mm/h
- CRP $\quad$ < 0.5
- Us & Es and LFTs normal
- C3 $\quad$ 0.38 $\quad$ (0.55–1.2 g/l)
- C4 $\quad$ 0.1 $\quad$ (0.2–0.5 g/l)
- IgG $\quad$ 20.5 $\quad$ (7.0–18.0 g/l)
- IgM $\quad$ 2.0 $\quad$ (0.4–2.5 g/l)
- IgA $\quad$ 3.2 $\quad$ (0.8–4 g/l)
- ANA: $\quad$ 1/1280 fine speckled pattern

- Rheumatoid factor: negative
- Double stranded DNA: 128 (normal < 50)
- Antibodies to extractable nuclear antigens:

  anti-sm   positive
  anti-ro ⎫
  la   ⎬ negative
  RNP   ⎭
  Jo-1

- Direct Coomb's test (DAT): negative
- Antibody to anticardiolipin antibody: negative
- Clotting screen: normal.

Follow-up outpatient appointment one month later.

Doctor: How have you been feeling since I last saw you?

Patient: About the same. Really tired all the time and my joints still hurt.

Doctor: Any new symptoms?

Patient: No.

Doctor: And has the rash come back?

Patient: I've had some spots on my chest off and on, but nothing else since I last saw you.

Doctor: Well, the results of your tests are back. These confirm that the problems you've been having are due to a condition called systemic lupus erythematosus, or lupus for short, which you may remember I explained was a possibility last time. In this condition the body's immune system turns traitor,[15] so instead of fighting bugs, which it is supposed to be doing, it starts attacking us. It can attack different organs and it's likely that your immune system has been attacking your joints and your skin, causing the problems you've been having with pain and stiffness and rashes. There's no evidence that any other organs have become involved. It also has general effects which explain why you've been feeling so unwell. For example, tiredness is very common.

Patient: Is there any treatment?

Doctor: We can't get rid of the underlying condition, but we can help with controlling the disease, and helping the symptoms you've been having. I would like to start you on a drug which has been shown to be helpful for joint pain, rashes and the tiredness. It is called hydroxy-chloroquine. It is a tablet to be taken twice a day. It doesn't usually cause any side-effects. However, I would like you to have an eye test. This is because a related drug, called chloroquine, that was used before hydroxy-chloroquine, did occasionally cause damage to the back of the eye. The drug was used in far bigger doses than we use now, and there doesn't seem to be the same problem with hydroxy-chloroquine. However, until we are certain that the new drug doesn't cause the same problem, we are advising people to see an eye doctor, who will explain how you can monitor to ensure that your eyes are not being damaged. I will also give you a stronger pain killer. It is called Voltarol. You can take it for the joint pain and stiffness when you want to, up to a maximum of three tablets a day. It is best taken with food. The commonest side-effect is heartburn.[16]

Patient: What's going to happen in the future?

Doctor: At this stage it's too early to say. I'd like to see you regularly in the clinic to see how you're doing. Some people develop problems with different organs and we will need to monitor you. Hopefully, the tablets I am giving you should make you feel considerably better. Do you have any other questions?

Patient: No. It's all a bit of a shock.

Doctor: Yes and there's a lot to take in,[17] but I'd like to see you again shortly to go through a few more things and we can go over[18] anything that I haven't made clear today. Do write down any questions you have in the meantime, so that we can cover everything you're worried about.

Patient: Thank you, doctor.

Explanations

1. **kid:** child.
2. **yeah:** yes.
3. **first thing:** early morning.
4. **knackered:** exhausted.
5. **been off your food:** loss of appetite.

6. **half a stone:** seven pounds in weight.
7. **blotchy:** patches of discoloration on skin.
8. **for ages:** for a long time.
9. **loads:** a lot.
10. **contacts:** contact lenses.
11. **miscarriages:** spontaneous abortion.
12. **Gran:** grandmother.
13. **waterworks:** bladder.
14. **periods:** menstruation.
15. **turns traitor:** fails to help.
16. **heartburn:** pyrosis.
17. **take in:** information to absorb, understand.
18. **go over:** discuss.

22. Woman, aged 25

Doctor: When did the present attack begin?

Patient: It started on Christmas Eve[1] and I couldn't get the tablets. I had to keep going to the loo.[2] I only passed a small amount and it was stinging. There was a lot of blood with clots.

Doctor: Where was the pain?

Patient: Down here. (suprapubic)

Doctor: Did you have a pain in the loin?

Patient: No.

Doctor: Did you have a fever with it?

Patient: No, but I did last time.

Doctor: How long does it last?

Patient: When I get the tablets it goes in a few days.

Doctor: Do you take Septrin?

Patient: Yes, most of the time Septrin and some green medicine.[3]

Doctor: In between attacks do you have to go often to the lavatory?

Patient: Yes. I can't wait.

Doctor: How long have you had this trouble?

Patient: Since I had my children.

Doctor: How many have you?

Patient: Two: five and six. There's only eleven months between them.

Doctor: Did you have any trouble in pregnancy?

Patient: No. It's been worse since my second.

Doctor: When you cough, strain, sneeze, does your water come away from you?

Patient: Yes.

Doctor: Did you have a difficult and long labour?

Patient: No.

Doctor: Did you have a forceps delivery?

Patient: Yes.

Doctor: Do you have to get up in the night?

Patient: No.

Doctor: Can you think of anything else that brings it on?[4]

Patient: I wonder if it is the coil.[5]

Doctor: How long have you used it?

Patient: Three years. When they put it in, I had it[6] straight away after.

Doctor: Have you had it changed?

Patient: No.

Doctor: Are you under the Family Planning Clinic?

Patient: Yes.

Doctor: Why do you use the coil instead of the pill?[7]

Patient: I got migraine with the pill.

Doctor: Do you still get migraine?

Patient: Very occasionally.

Doctor: Do you think there is any connection between the attacks and intercourse?

Patient: No.

Doctor: What about your weight?

Patient: It's steady.

Doctor: Your appetite?

Patient: It's very poor. It always has been.

Doctor: Your bowels?

Patient: Regular.

Doctor: And how are your periods?

Patient: I lose four days every twenty-eight days.

Doctor: Have you ever been anaemic?

Patient: No.

Doctor: Do you smoke?

Patient: Thirty a day.

Doctor: Do you drink?

Patient: Only at the weekends.

Doctor: Have you had any other illnesses?

Patient: No.

Doctor: Did you ever have this trouble as a child?

Patient: Yes, when I was about five. I didn't tell anybody.

Doctor: Did you wet your bed later than is normal?

Patient: No.

Doctor: Is there anyone in your family with water trouble?

Patient: Yes. My mother has it. She's been on tablets for nine years. When she stops taking them, it comes back.

Doctor: Is there anyone else with it?

Patient: Yes. My sister has it three or four times a year. It started after her first child.

Doctor: Any other family?

Patient: I have a father and brother.

Doctor: Are they all right?

Patient: Yes.

Doctor: Well, we must have your kidney and bladder X-rayed. If there is nothing wrong there, we must put you on tablets. Strip down to your underpants and cover yourself with a blanket.

The doctor gave the following instructions during the clinical examination:

- I'm just going to take your blood pressure.
- Stare up at the ceiling. (Examines fundi with ophthalmoscope.)
- I'll just feel under your arms. (Palpates for lymph nodes.)
- I'm going to listen to your heart now. Take a deep breath in and out.
- Breathe through your mouth. (Auscultates chest.)

    – Sit forward. I'm going to tap your back now. (Percussion of spine and renal areas for loin tenderness.)

    – I'm going to feel your neck. (Palpates for lymph nodes.)

Patient: I had some lumps in my neck.

Doctor: Did you have a sore throat?

Patient: Yes.

Doctor: Probably a little gland came up. Let's feel your tummy. (Palpates abdomen.) Lie back on my hand. Does that hurt you at the front or back? (Palpates each loin bimanually.)

Patient: Back.

Doctor: Now your legs. Bend your knees. (Elicits knee jerks.) I'm going to tickle your feet. (Elicits plantar response.) I want to examine your back passage.[8] Please take off your pants. Turn over and curl yourself into a ball with your bottom[9] right over the edge of the couch. This is a bit uncomfortable. Tell me if there is any tender spot. (Performs rectal examination.)

Patient: No.

Doctor: Nurse will wipe the lubricant off your bottom. I'm going to take a drop of your blood now. I can't find anything wrong in examining you but we must obviously look into this further to see if there is any cause for these repeated infections. Make an appointment for a kidney X-ray. You can get dressed now.

Clinical notes

    – Thin long-limbed healthy girl

    – Not anaemic

O/E

    – CVS   P 80

                  Ht not enlarged

                  Ht sounds √

                  BP $\dfrac{130}{90}$

    – Fundi   0

    – Chest   √

- No glands
- Abd.   Slight tenderness over sigmoid colon
- No renal masses
- PR   NAD
- CNS   NAD

Investigations
- IVP
- MSU
- CXR
- FBC
- U and E
- RBS

Explanations
1. **Christmas Eve:** December 24th.
2. **had to keep going to the loo:** had to go frequently to the lavatory to pass water (but it can also mean because of diarrhoea).
3. **green medicine:** potassium citrate known as pot.cit.
4. **brings it on:** causes it.
5. **the coil:** intrauterine contraceptive device.
6. **it:** the urinary trouble.
7. **the pill:** oral contraceptive.
8. **back passage:** rectum.
9. **bottom:** buttocks.

Letter to GP from Consultant

Whittington Hospital
Highgate Hill
London N19

5 January 2002

Dr S Popplewell
10 York Rise
London N6

Dear Dr Popplewell

Pamela Harvey (F) 7 6 77, 53 Park Close, London, N6

Thank you for referring this patient who gives an interesting history of frequent urinary infections occurring about every 4 months since marriage 6 years ago. However, there is no clear-cut relation to intercourse nor is there any other precipitating factor. Each attack seems to respond rapidly to treatment and there is nothing to suggest permanent renal damage. There is an interesting family history with her mother and sister having similar symptoms. Her mother is on long-term prophylaxis and she has relapses if she ever stops taking the tablets.

I could not find any significant signs on general and rectal examination apart from slight tenderness over the sigmoid colon. I have ordered IVP and other relevant investigations to exclude any underlying cause.

Should nothing be found, it might be advisable to treat her in the same way as her mother with long-term chemoprophylaxis.

Yours sincerely

David Layton
Consultant Physician

23. Woman, aged 54

Referred by her GP with a history of low back pain.

Doctor: Well, Mrs Cairns come and sit down. Your GP says you've had low back pain for many years.

Patient: Yes indeed. I've had it for twenty years. It started after I had my son.

Doctor: How many children have you?

Patient: Just the one son.

Doctor: When do you get the pain?

Patient: It's worse after walking.

Doctor: Does it spread down your legs?

Patient: No. It's not a bad pain but it goes on. I'm worried I might get like my mother. She was very stooped and lost height.

Doctor: How old was she when this happened?

Patient: In her late seventies. She had brittle bone disease[1] and eventually broke her hip and died. I'm worried I might get the same thing.

Doctor: Does the pain wake you up at night?

Patient: No.

Doctor: When did your periods stop?

Patient: I had to have a hysterectomy when I was forty. Then I got hot flushes when I was about forty-two.

Doctor: Have you ever broken a leg or arm?

Patient: No. It's just the back ache that worries me.

Doctor: What about eating? Do you have a healthy diet?

Patient: Yes I think so – I have a mixed diet and plenty of cheese and fruit. I don't drink much milk though – about a quarter of a pint a day.

Doctor: Do you drink?[2]

Patient: Mmm. About half a bottle of wine a day with my meals.

Doctor: And smoke?

Patient: Not at all.

Doctor: Your GP says you had an overactive thyroid when you were twenty-five, had an operation and are now on thyroxine replacement tablets.

Patient: Yes that's right.

Doctor: Have you ever been on HRT?[3]

Patient: Never.

Doctor: Well, I'd like to examine you. Slip off all your clothes except your pants and bra and lie on the couch.

Clinical notes

O/E
- BP 150/90
- NAD
- No deformity of spine
- Breasts normal
- Clinically euthyroid

Conclusion
- Early menopause
- Previous thyrotoxicosis
- Slightly raised BP
- Risk of premature osteoporosis

Investigations
- Bone density scan
- Serum TSH level
- Full blood count
- Plasma, urea + electrolytes
- Calcium + liver function tests

Doctor: Well, Mrs Cairns I can't find anything wrong with you except a slightly raised blood pressure. You did, however, have an early menopause and thyrotoxicosis previously so this does give a risk of premature osteoporosis. I'd like you to have some tests done before I see you again. I want you to have a bone density scan.

Patient: What does it entail?

Doctor: It is a low-powered X-ray scan of your spine and hip. It takes only five minutes and is not harmful.

Return visit:

Doctor: Hello, Mrs Cairns. Come and sit down. Well I've got the results of the tests we did and the bone density T score is −2.9. By definition anything worse than −2.5 is osteoporosis. All the other tests were normal. Your blood pressure was 145 over 80 when taken again which is normal.

Patient: So can anything be done about the osteoporosis?

Doctor: Yes, we can put you on HRT for about ten years.

Patient: Could it cause cancer?

Doctor: There's no definite evidence of an increase of breast cancer if the patient has HRT for up to ten years. But there is a big reduction in the risk of having a heart attack. If you don't like the idea of HRT an alternative is a bisphosphonate. This protects the bone but has no other advantages.

Patient: All right. Well I'll have HRT if you advise that.

Doctor: I do. I'll write to your GP to start you on Premarin. Apart from that, drink more milk, take gentle exercise and reduce your alcohol intake. Come back in a year's time for a bone density test.

Patient: Thank you doctor.

Explanations
1. **brittle bone disease:** osteoporosis.
2. **Do you drink?:** this means 'Do you drink alcohol?'.
3. **HRT:** hormone replacement therapy.

24. Man, aged 45

Doctor: Good morning Mr Carter. I'm Dr Hartley. Dr Walters has asked me to see you and has sent me a letter. Shall we go through things[1] together? How old are you?

Patient: Forty-five.

Doctor: Tell me how long you've been unwell.

Patient: Well, I've had a sore mouth for six months and I started losing weight four months ago.

Doctor: Any other problems?

Patient: Well, I've been sweating, especially at night.

Doctor: How bad is the sweating?

Patient: Bad enough to soak[2] the sheets.

Doctor: Have you had a cough?

Patient: No.

Doctor: Have you ever had TB or been in contact with anyone with TB?

Patient: One of my friends died of AIDS and he had TB.

Doctor: Was that ordinary TB?

Patient: I'm not certain but I don't think it was the resistant TB that was discussed on TV the other night. I know that it wasn't MAIC because one of my friends had that and he had different tablets.

Doctor: I see. Would you consider yourself at risk from HIV?

Patient: Well, I've been very careful over the last three years but before that I used to be quite promiscuous.[3]

Doctor: Have you ever had any sexually transmitted diseases, like gonorrhoea?

Patient: Yes, I had gonorrhoea ten years ago. I was treated for it at St Mary's Hospital.

Doctor: Have you ever had herpes?

Patient: No.

Doctor: Were you having sex with your friend who died of AIDS?

Patient: No, but we did have a joint lover.

Doctor: Have you been worrying about being infected with HIV?

Patient: Yes, when I started to lose weight and got the night sweats. I knew they were the same symptoms my friend got.

Doctor: Have you discussed this properly with anyone else?

Patient: I talked a bit about it with Dr Walters but he said it was best to see you.

Doctor: Have you been in contact with the Terence Higgins Trust[4] or any other voluntary bodies?

Patient: No.

Doctor: Is there anything else you'd like to tell me at this stage?

Patient: No. I've no other problems.

Doctor: Can you tell me if you are taking any medicine of any kind?

Patient: I've been taking live yoghurt because I thought I had thrush[5] in my mouth.

Doctor: Do you smoke or drink?

Patient: I don't smoke and I only have alcohol occasionally.

Doctor: Well, I'd like to examine you.

Clinical examination

Doctor: You have sore patches on the corner of your mouth. How long have you had them?

Patient: For six months.

Doctor: So you still have thrush in your mouth. Has the yoghurt helped?

Patient: I think so.

Doctor: Have you noticed any skin rashes?

Patient: Yes, my face has gone dry. There's also a patch under my arm.

Doctor: This rash around your anus looks like herpes. How long have you had it?

Patient: A month.

Doctor: You can get dressed now.

After patient is dressed:

Doctor: Your GP wonders whether you want to be tested for HIV. How do you feel about it?

Patient: I'm very frightened. Do you think some of my problems could be related to AIDS?

Doctor: Yes, I'm afraid that some of the skin changes and the candida and the soreness at the side of your mouth are commonly seen in people who are HIV positive.

Patient: Yes, I was afraid you'd say that. Well, we might as well get on[6] with the test then.

Doctor: Well, I want to discuss some other issues first. Do you understand the difference between AIDS and HIV positive?

Patient: Not really.

Doctor: The antibody only tells us that you have at some time been infected by the virus. It does not tell us anything about what is happening to you now or what will happen in the future. It is very important to know how you would handle[7] this information if it comes back positive. Who would support you?

Patient: I don't know. My parents don't even know I'm gay.[8] I wouldn't want them to know. My twin brother knows I'm not very well. He might be willing to help me.

Doctor: Would you like to speak to a colleague of mine who is very helpful as a counsellor?

Patient: Yes.

Doctor: I could also give you the phone number of the Terence Higgins Trust and other organisations.

Patient: I'm not really interested as I'm not into the gay scene, strange as it may seem.

Doctor: I'd like to talk to you about things like mortgages and life insurance. Do you understand that if I take this blood test it could jeopardise your chances of a life insurance and getting a mortgage?

Patient: Well, I didn't know that but it doesn't worry me. I'd like to have the blood test.

Doctor: If I do the blood test today I could see you to give you the result tomorrow. If it is positive we will take a second sample to make sure that there has been no error.

Patient: Could you post me the result?

Doctor: I'll want you to come back. We never give this information except person-to-person even if it is negative.

Clinical notes

– O/E   Eczematous rash round nose and mouth/angular cheilosis.

Red area 10 cm in 1. axilla.

No other rash except dandruff in scalp.

– BP $\dfrac{130}{80}$

- P   90
- Chest   clear
- Abdomen   NAD
- Soft nodes up to 1 cm diameter both sides of neck and both groins.
- Perianal skin: reddened, inflamed,? herpetic.

Return visit 24 hours later:

Doctor: Good morning Mr Carter. Come and sit down.

Patient: I've brought my brother with me.

Doctor: Good. How've you been?

Patient: Worse. My brother thinks I should tell you about the 'flu symptoms I've had for the last week or so.

Doctor: Oh yes. I think that's important too. Why didn't you tell me about this yesterday?

Patient: It didn't seem so important.

Doctor: Well, tell me about it now. Have you a cough?

Patient: Yes.

Doctor: Do you bring up any sputum?

Patient: No.

Doctor: Have you had any fevers?

Patient: Yes and bad sweats. I had one coming in the car just now and I was absolutely drenched.[9]

Doctor: Do you get out of breath?

Patient: Oh yes. I can't walk upstairs as easily as I could. I notice if I take a deep breath it makes me cough.

Doctor: Could you do that now? (Patient takes deep breath and coughs.) I want to listen to your chest. (Auscultates chest.) Good. That's clear. I'd like to see how far you can walk upstairs. Let's go into the passage. (Patient walks up 15 steps and is then gasping for breath. Returns to room.)

Doctor: So, you are much less fit than you were two months ago?

Patient: Yes, three or four weeks ago I could have climbed much further.

Doctor: Right. I would like you to go for an X-ray now. Are you worried that this is PCP?

Patient: What's PCP?

Doctor: I'm sorry. It is pneumocystis pneumonia.

Patient: Was my blood test positive? Do I have AIDS?

Doctor: I'm afraid you probably do.

Brother: Is there any treatment for it?

Doctor: Yes, we would admit your brother and start him on treatment with an antibiotic called co-trimoxazole which we will start intravenously. Later on he may be able to take it in tablet form at home.

Brother: I have heard about some new drugs that are very good – something called triple therapy.

Doctor: Yes, there are lots of exciting new drugs and I will discuss all of these with you but the first step is to confirm the PCP and to treat that.

X-ray showed reticular nodular shadowing consistent with PCP. Patient admitted. Started on treatment which proved beneficial.

Explanations

1. **go through:** discuss.
2. **to soak:** wet completely.
3. **to be promiscuous:** to have casual sex relations with many people.
4. **Terence Higgins Trust:** this is a major charitable organisation offering advice and help to HIV positive people.
5. **thrush:** candida.
6. **get on with:** do the test now.
7. **handle:** react to.
8. **gay:** homosexual.
9. **drenched:** wet completely.

25. Woman, aged 59

Doctor: I see you have had several attacks of influenza. Anything else?

Patient: I've had dizziness and I've been sick.[1]

Doctor: When did this start?

Patient: Two months ago.

Doctor: How often are the attacks?

Patient: Nearly every day.

Doctor: How long do they last?

Patient: Some last all day, some a couple of hours.

Doctor: Does anything bring on these attacks?

Patient: No.

Doctor: Will you describe one of these attacks?

Patient: It starts with a headache – a throbbing headache. My eyes start running. I can't touch them, they are so sore.[2] And then the whole house goes round. Then it goes dark.

Doctor: Do you see flashing lights?

Patient: No.

Doctor: When you say you go dizzy, what do you mean?[3]

Patient: I feel I'll fall over and the room spins[4] round. If I go to bed, the bed goes round.

Doctor: When you move, do you stagger?[5]

Patient: I'm too scared to move.[6]

Doctor: Have you noticed anything else?

Patient: I cough a lot.

Doctor: Do you bring anything up?[7]

Patient: No.

Doctor: Is your hearing affected? Do you have buzzing[8] or ringing noises?

Patient: Yes.

Doctor: In both ears?

Patient: Yes.

Doctor: When you go to bed, do you sleep?

Patient: I just lie and it goes off[9] within a few hours.

Doctor: Have you ever woken up like this?

Patient: No. It is always in the day.

Doctor: Does movement of the head cause it?

Patient: No.

Doctor: If you suddenly get up out of a chair does it start?

Patient: No.

Doctor: How long have you been diabetic?

Patient: Four years.

Doctor: Any other serious illness?

Patient: I had my gall bladder removed.

Doctor: Anything else?

Patient: I had VD nine years ago. I was in hospital for three weeks and had a course of injections.

The doctor gave the following instructions during the clinical examination:

Doctor: Take a deep breath in and hold your breath. Close your eyes gently. Not too tight. Look up to the ceiling. Hold your arms out. Are your bowels all right?

Patient: Yes.

Doctor: No trouble with your water?

Patient: No.

Doctor: Your periods finished some years ago?

Patient: Yes. Four years ago.

Doctor: Well, there doesn't seem anything seriously wrong with you. I'd like you to have some X-rays though and a blood test.

Explanations

1. **dizziness:** vertigo. **been sick:** vomited.
2. **my eyes start running:** watering. **sore:** tender, irritating.
3. **dizzy:** vertigo.
4. **spins:** moves round, rotates.
5. **stagger:** move unsteadily.
6. **scared:** frightened.
7. **bring anything up:** bring up sputum, expectorate.
8. **buzzing:** like the sound made by insects.
9. **goes off:** stops.

26. Woman, aged 69

Patient complaining of severe pain in right arm and right leg. Follow-up clinic.

Doctor: How've you been, Mrs Cooper?

Patient: Terrible, terrible.

Doctor: I'm sorry. Let me see. How long is it since I saw you?

Patient: It's three months. I had two lots of physiotherapy but it gave me terrible pain.

Doctor: Did we do an X-ray?

Patient: Yes, of my neck.

Doctor: Yes, here it is. You've got a bit of arthritis. How did you get on with the tablets?[1]

Patient: Oh, I can't take them. They made me feel sick.[2] The only ones I can take are paracetamol.

Doctor: Well, take off your clothes so I can see your shoulder and neck.

O/E:

Doctor: Is the pain on all the time or only when you walk?

Patient: Nearly all the time.

Doctor: Put your arms above your head. Does that hurt?

Patient: No.

Doctor: Is that tender?

Patient: No.

Doctor: Is the pain in the joints worse in the mornings?

Patient: Yes.

Doctor: Any tingling in the hands and feet?

Patient: A little in the feet.

Doctor: What about the waterworks?[3]

Patient: I go more than I used to.[4]

Doctor: Do you have full control?

Patient: Yes.

Doctor: Bowels?

Patient: All right.

Doctor: Do your feet feel they're not really on the ground?

Patient: Sometimes.

Doctor: Let me look at your feet. Just relax. Can you feel me touching you? Does that feel hot or cold?

Patient: Cold.

Doctor: Do your feet feel cold all the time?

Patient: Yes.

Doctor: Hold the leg up and push down. Press down as hard as you can.

Now relax the leg. Let your legs go loose and relax. Let your foot drop. I'm going to scratch the bottom of your feet. Does it feel the same both sides? Does that feel hot or cold?

Patient: Yes. They feel cold.

Doctor: What do you feel there?

Patient: Tingling.

Doctor: Sit up. I'll look at your neck. The pain is there, is it?

Patient: Yes.

Doctor: If I touch you here, does that feel normal?

Patient: Yes.

Doctor: Well, there's nothing wrong with the nerves. All the nerves are working perfectly well. But maybe one of the nerves is irritated. Which joints give you most trouble?

Patient: My arm.

Doctor: Well, what I could do would be to give you an injection. It often helps to relieve joint pain. How do you feel about that?

Patient: Could it help the pain?

Doctor: Yes. Shall I try? It's up to you.[5] It won't do any harm. It's just like a blood test.

Patient: Yes, I'll have it.

Doctor gives patient an injection of steroid into the shoulder joint.

Doctor: I'll put a plaster on. That will be a bit sore. Take a paracetamol. You should feel better tomorrow. You can get dressed now. I'll see you in six weeks.

Explanations

1. **How did you get on with the tablets?:** Were the drugs beneficial?
2. **feel sick:** have nausea.
3. **waterworks:** bladder.
4. **I go more than I used to:** I pass more water nowadays.
5. **It's up to you:** you must decide.

27. Woman, aged 27

Psychiatric unit.

Doctor: You've been in the Medical Ward recently. How are you feeling now?

Patient: Oh, better.

Doctor: What exactly was the trouble?

Patient: I began to feel dizzy[1] and then I got palpitations and felt limp.[2] It lasted about an hour. I woke up and my legs were heavy. It has eased off a bit.[3] I only get one a week now[4] and since I left hospital I've had none for three weeks.

Doctor: When did all this start?

Patient: Last October. I went to my GP[5] and he gave me some Valium.[6] It wasn't any good. I began to lose my nerve[7] in the street. I daren't cross the road because my legs went heavy. I was working full-time in the day and coming home and cooking dinner, cleaning and I suppose it was all too much.

Doctor: What was the dizzy feeling like?

Patient: I felt like toppling.[8]

Doctor: Did you feel unsteady or were things going round you?

Patient: I felt shifty[9] as if I was moving rather than actual things moving.

Doctor: Did things seem normal around you?

Patient: Oh yes. Only I felt shifty, trembly, unsteady.

Doctor: Did it come on first at work?

Patient: It came on first one day when I was coming home from work.

Doctor: Did it last long?

Patient: No, but I lost my nerve crossing the street.

Doctor: What happened then?

Patient: I got palpitations and these attacks. I began to go limp[10] and I went to my doctor[11] and he referred me here.

Doctor: Did you notice that any particular thing started an attack?

Patient: It was usually at night, when I was coming home from

shopping or coming back from the launderette[12] or
something like that.

Doctor: How long have you been married?

Patient: One year and four months.

Doctor: Have you any children?

Patient: No. I'd hoped to start a family[13] but nothing's happened.
I began crying at my periods[14] and I felt disheartened.

Doctor: Was that why you felt worse at night before going to bed?

Patient: I don't know. I've had arthritis and working and cooking
— everything's been too much for me.

Doctor: What do you mean by palpitations?

Patient: I feel my heart banging and I get breathless.

Doctor: Are you puffed[15] during attacks?

Patient: No.

Doctor: You say your arms and legs are heavy?[16]

Patient: Yes, I can't lift anything.

Doctor: Have you noticed anything else?

Patient: I have a tingling[17] sense in my muscles.

Doctor: How long have you been out of hospital?

Patient: Nearly three weeks.

Doctor: Have you any idea why you haven't had these attacks?

Patient: I've been trying to help myself. The gynaecologist gave
me a temperature chart. I'm on a diet and I feel a bit
more contented.

Doctor: Do you sleep well?

Patient: Yes.

Doctor: How's your appetite? Good?

Patient: Yes. I've been trying to cut down.[18]

Doctor: What about your parents?

Patient: My father died when I was eleven of leukaemia.

Doctor: Do you remember much about him?

Patient: Vaguely.[19] My Mum and Dad used to scream at each
other and I had nightmares about it. My Mum's 65 now
and she had an operation on her hip for arthritis. She
lives in a flat with no lift so she can never go out.

Doctor: How did you get on when you lived at home?[20]

Patient: We used to argue when I was younger about cleaning and things.

Doctor: Have you any brothers and sisters?

Patient: I have two brothers and one sister.

Doctor: Where do you come in?

Patient: I'm the baby by five years.

Doctor: So you weren't all that happy when you were growing up?

Patient: No.

Doctor: Did your mother ever remarry?

Patient: No.

Doctor: How did she manage?[21]

Patient: She managed all right.

Doctor: Did she work?

Patient: She worked for a bit[22] but she's very independent.

Doctor: How about school?

Patient: I didn't like school.

Doctor: What about work? What did you do?

Patient: I worked in an office typing. It was all right at the beginning but I got fed up.[23]

Doctor: So you've not been happy recently?

Patient: No. Last year I was a clerical assistant but I had to give it up.[24]

Doctor: What would you really like to do?

Patient: Well, I'm very limited.

Doctor: By what?

Patient: By this arthritis in my arms.

Doctor: Well, what would you like to do?

Patient: I'd like to be on a switchboard. You see, people in offices worry me. They get me down.[25]

Doctor: In what way?

Patient: Well, I work hard and some others do no work. It gets me down.

Doctor: What about your husband? How old is he?

Patient: He's six years older than me.

Doctor: What does he do?

Patient: He's a steel fitter in building. He's self-employed now.

Doctor: Is that regular?

Patient: Yes, it is now but he was out of work when we first got married.

Doctor: How do you get on?[26]

Patient: Oh, all right. We have our little tiffs[27] but nothing much.

Doctor: What do you have tiffs about?

Patient: Oh, sometimes I get tired and he says things should be done. I think he'd like everything done nicely but I get tired.

Doctor: Does he have very high standards?

Patient: Well, we live in a basement flat. It gets very dirty. I try to scrub the kitchen floor and clean the window and everything but it gets dirty again quickly so I get disheartened. I wrote to the housing people[28] but they asked for a doctor's letter. My doctor refused to give me a letter. We have no bath. Then I have this arm. It slows me down and then in two days' time after all the cleaning, it's dirty again. We have no cupboard space either so everything is in boxes all over the place.

Doctor: When did you see the gynaecologist?

Patient: Yesterday.

Doctor: What did she say?

Patient: She told me to carry on with the temperature chart. My husband has had a test and I'm to come back in two months.

Doctor: Has this always been your big thing[29] to be a mother?

Patient: Yes. You see I used to take ten minutes to do a job but it takes me an hour now with these arms.

Doctor: How long have you had arthritis?

Patient: Four years.

Doctor: Is the main trouble the tiredness in the arms?

Patient: Yes. I want something to take my mind off myself. That's why I want a baby.

Doctor: Why have you given up doing things? Because you are slow?

Patient: Yes, and because I lack confidence. If I do things I think they are not good enough. I know it's the wrong attitude but I can't help it.

Doctor: Have you always lacked confidence?

Patient: No. I used to go swimming and take my clothes off. Now I want to cover up.

Doctor: Why?

Patient: My arms are not straight. I want to cover up and go into my little shell.[30]

Doctor: What do you do all day?

Patient: I tidy up, make the dinner, watch telly.[31] That's me.

Doctor: You'd feel a lot better if you did more you know. What about at night?

Patient: Well, my husband comes home tired and he doesn't want to do much. I go to bingo[32] once a week. My husband goes to a man's club once a week.

Doctor: Have you any friends?

Patient: No. I have one who's having a baby in three weeks.

Doctor: I think it's a great mistake to get out of touch with people and get so bored.

Patient: I used to enjoy visiting people but now I feel restless and want to go home.

Doctor: It is important to build up contacts and interests. There is nothing seriously wrong with your nerves. These attacks are nervous in origin but they are just attacks of anxiety. You are anxious about your illness, anxious about your house, anxious about not having a baby. Yet at the same time your life is becoming more and more restricted into a home that doesn't please you at all. You don't need any special treatment. You've already worked out[33] some of this for yourself.

Patient: Well, I was worried about myself.

Doctor: I think the most important thing is to try and deal with some of the aspects of the increasing boredom in your life.

Patient: The housing is the main thing. I've never had a decent place. At my mother's we had bugs in the bed. I've saved up money for furniture but it's so damp and cold it's no good buying new things. I sit with my dressing gown on in front of the gas fire I'm so cold.

Doctor: I'll write to your doctor and see if he'll write to the Town Hall. You would be more likely to get new housing on medical grounds than emotional ones. But you must try to widen your circle of friends.

Patient: (breaking down)[34] Well, I used to go to a friend but she said I must get a job or else my husband will think he's married to an invalid.[35]

Doctor: Well, sometimes friends can say things that hurt. You must have many friends. Keep the contacts open. Then you can compare what all your friends say. It is very difficult to get houses in this area I know. I'll write to your doctor to reconsider it.

Patient: Yes. My husband would like a bath when he comes home dirty from work but all he has is a little bowl. Do you think I should see this friend even if she says these things to me? Perhaps she didn't mean it like that...

Doctor: Yes. See your old friends and make new ones and try not to take everything to heart so much.[36] Would you like to come and talk to me again in a couple of weeks' time?

Patient: All right. Thank you Doctor.

Explanations

1. **to feel dizzy:** experience vertigo.
2. **felt limp:** felt weak.
3. **eased off:** became less frequent.
4. **one a week:** one attack of these symptoms.
5. **GP:** General Practitioner, formerly called Family Doctor. Patients are referred to hospital doctors by their GPs.
6. **Valium:** a tranquilizer.
7. **to lose my nerve:** to lose confidence.
8. **toppling:** falling over, collapsing.
9. **shifty:** unsteady (note: this is an unusual use of the word).
10. **to go limp:** to feel weak.
11. **my doctor:** my GP, the doctor I am registered with.

12. **the launderette:** a public laundry with coin-operated washing machines.
13. **to start a family:** to become pregnant.
14. **periods:** menstruation.
15. **puffed:** out of breath, breathless.
16. a statement-question, see Case History 17, note 7.
17. **tingling:** prickling, like pins and needles.
18. **to cut down:** to reduce food intake.
19. **vaguely:** not clearly.
20. **how did you get on?:** what was your relationship like?
21. **how did she manage?:** what did she live on?
22. **for a bit:** for a short time.
23. **fed up:** bored, discontented.
24. **give it up:** stop doing that job.
25. **they get me down:** they upset me.
26. **how do you get on:** what is your relationship like?
27. **a tiff:** a slight quarrel.
28. **the housing people:** the Housing Department of the Local Authority.
29. **your big thing:** the most important thing, what you want most.
30. **go into my little shell:** hide myself.
31. **telly:** television.
32. **bingo:** popular gambling game held in public rooms.
33. **worked out:** found out, realised.
34. **breaking down:** bursting into tears.
35. **invalid:** someone who is always ill.
36. **try not to take things to heart:** try not to be too hurt by people's remarks.

28. Woman, aged 22

Doctor: Hello, Miss Wells. Please come and sit down. I am Miss Moore, the Consultant, and I have read your GP's referral letter which details your past history of endometriosis. I wonder if I

could start off by asking you some questions. How old are you now?

Patient: Twenty-two.

Doctor: Are you married?

Patient: No, but I am living with my partner.

Doctor: Have you ever been pregnant?

Patient: No.

Doctor: When was your last cervical smear?

Patient: This was done when I went to see my GP about three months ago.

Doctor: Do you know the result?

Patient: Yes, it was normal.

Doctor: Now I gather that you had some pelvic pain. Would you like to describe to me what the problem is?

Patient: It started in February of this year when I was admitted to another hospital with acute pain in the left side of my tummy.[1] I had this pain for some time and it usually started a few days before my period and then seemed to settle at the end of my period. Since February it has got really bad and it would not go away, so I was admitted as an emergency to the hospital. The Consultant there performed a laparoscopy and it showed endometriosis behind my womb[2] and on my left ovary. After that, he suggested that I should take the pill[3] without a break, but the pain did not get better at all and so he started me on progesterone tablets, but these made me feel horrible and made me put on[4] weight and feel bloated[5] and I developed acne. Also the pain was no better and I was also having pain during sexual intercourse. The Consultant therefore readmitted me in May of this year and he performed another laparoscopy and treated the endometriosis with a diathermy. After that, I was much better and the pain almost completely went until August of this year when it restarted. It has slowly been getting worse, and again, as in the beginning, the left side of my tummy hurts just before my periods, but now it is starting to be painful again at different parts of the month and it really hurts when we make love particularly in certain positions.

Doctor: May I ask you if your periods are regular?

Patient: Yes, regular because I am still taking the pill with a week's break.

Doctor: Do you have any bleeding in between periods or after sexual intercourse?

Patient: No.

Doctor: Do you have any discharge? Are your periods heavy?

Patient: No, they are fine as long as[6] I take the pill. They become really heavy when I don't take the pill.

Doctor: How old were you when your periods started?

Patient: Thirteen. Then my periods were really painful and heavy.

Doctor: When was your last period?

Patient: About three weeks ago.

Doctor: Now I would like to ask you some more general questions. Do you have any problems passing water?

Patient: No.

Doctor: How about your bowels – are they regular?

Patient: Yes.

Doctor: Do you have them opened every day?

Patient: Yes.

Doctor: Do you ever experience any pain when you pass your motions?

Patient: No.

Doctor: In the past, have you had any serious illnesses?

Patient: No, I only had my tonsils removed.

Doctor: Do you have any allergies?

Patient: No.

Doctor: Do you take any tablets apart from the pill?

Patient: No, I don't.

Doctor: Are there any problems in your family?

Patient: No, my mother and father and sisters are well.

Doctor: Do you smoke or drink much alcohol?

Patient: No I don't smoke and only drink alcohol at weekends.

Doctor: What do you do for a job?

Patient: I work for a charity organisation and my boyfriend has also just got a job, so we therefore moved to London recently, which is why I have transferred care from my previous Consultant.

Doctor: Right Miss Smith. I think it would be sensible to have a look at you and then we can chat about how to take things forward afterwards. Has anybody examined your breasts recently?

Patient: No. I do sometimes examine them myself, but I have not really had a breast examination.

Doctor: Right. Perhaps it would then be easiest if you take all your clothes off and put one of these blue gowns on behind these curtains here and put your clothes on the chair and there is a sheet you can cover yourself with. After you have undressed I will be with you in a minute.

Clinical Examination:

Doctor: May I have a look at your breasts please? Lift your arms up. Thank you. Your breasts feel normal and I can't detect any lumps. I would now like to examine your tummy and then do a vaginal examination. Do you feel any pain in your tummy at the moment?

Patient: Yes, I do have slight pain down here on the left.

Doctor: When did this pain start?

Patient: About two days ago, but my period is due and that's always when it is worse.

Doctor: I am going to examine your tummy now and if you could tell me where the pain is worst.

The next thing I would like to do is a vaginal examination. I am just going to warm up the speculum and then I will have a look at the neck of the womb and then also examine you internally with my hand. Could you please bend your knees and put your feet together and let your legs fall apart.

Are you comfortable?

Patient: Yes.

Doctor: Please tell me if I hurt you. I will try and be as gentle as possible. I am now introducing the speculum. Is this comfortable?

Patient: Yes.

Doctor: Good. The vagina looks normal and the neck of the womb looks very healthy. I will now take the speculum out and then examine you with my hands to see if I can feel where the pain is on the left side. Are you comfortable?

Patient: Yes, I am.

Doctor: Can you feel any pain at all on the right?

Patient: No, that's fine.

Doctor: I can now feel your uterus. Does that hurt?

Patient: No, that's not too bad.

Doctor: What about if I feel on the left side.

Patient: Oh yes, this really hurts.

Doctor: Well I can't feel any cysts, but you do seem to be very tender on that side. I have finished with the examination now. Would you like to get dressed and then we can talk about the next step. Please sit down again.

Miss Wells, from what you are telling me and also examining you today, it seems to me as if your endometriosis might have come back. Unfortunately, the only way we can tell for sure is by performing another laparoscopy. I don't think you have developed any cysts on your ovary, but to check for this we can do an ultrasound scan of the womb and the ovaries.

Patient: Since I was diagnosed as having endometriosis I have been doing a lot of reading and I am really worried that I have got the pain again. Also I would like to have some babies in the future and I think this may be difficult with the endometriosis. I wonder if it will ever go away because the pain is really getting me down.[9]

Doctor: Perhaps we could discuss one issue at a time. First of all, as regards your future fertility.

Yes, in some women there is an association between endometriosis and trying to have a baby and indeed for some women this is more difficult. Sometimes it can be explained by the fact that endometriosis can cause changes to the anatomy in that it can distort the tubes and the ovaries and cause adhesions, that is, tissue bands, but in other cases it seems very difficult to understand why a few spots of endometriosis should be associated with difficulties in having a baby. In other women we find endometriosis coincidentally at the time of an operation for something completely unrelated and these women will have had no problems in getting pregnant.

It is therefore difficult to know or even to tell you if you will definitely have problems getting pregnant. My advice perhaps would be not to wait too long once you and your partner have definitely decided that you want children, so that in case you do need help with getting pregnant this can be offered to you while you are still relatively young. I am sure you are aware that, for example, the success rate for IVF is much decreased in older women.

Does this all make sense to you and do you have any more questions about this issue?

Patient: No, I think I understand that, but I just hope I am not one of those women who will have problems having a baby, because my boyfriend and I would very much like to have a child in the near future.

Doctor: Addressing your second point and your worries about never being able to get rid of the endometriosis, I have certainly recently treated a young woman who has had very, very severe endometriosis and who is now completely free of the disease and indeed the symptoms. I think in your particular case it might be advisable to try taking the pill again continuously for the next three months so that you avoid menstruation. If this is successful then we may be able to prevent doing another laparoscopy and also we could keep you on the contraceptive pill for three months at a time and let you have a period every three months only which is perfectly safe and should be able to help resolve your endometriosis altogether. However, if the pain does not improve taking the pill continuously I think we do need to do another laparoscopy and consider further diathermy at the time, if appropriate, and then treat you with a drug which is called Zoladex (an LHRH analogue) which makes the body think that you are menopausal. Indeed this drug is extremely effective in treating endometriosis. You would have to take it for a maximum period of six months and, whilst you would suffer some menopausal symptoms during the treatment, it may well cure your endometriosis completely afterwards. Of course you would not have any periods while you are taking it.

Patient: I am not so sure about wanting to be menopausal and are there any long-term effects of this drug?

Doctor: No, there are not. The menopausal effects revert back to normal as soon as you stop the treatment.

Patient: Well I think at the moment I would like to avoid another laparoscopy.

Doctor: I perfectly understand that. Would you therefore accept taking the oral contraceptive pill continuously over the next three months?

Patient: I suppose that seems the best solution. I just hope it works[10] this time.

Doctor: Well, the pain is not nearly as bad as it was when you were seen in February and I believe that the pill therefore has a good chance of working if taken continuously. I would therefore suggest that I see you again in three months' time, but of course I would be very happy to see you earlier if your pain is not settling or indeed gets worse and then we will arrange for a repeat laparoscopy. I know you have read quite a lot, but we have produced a leaflet ourselves recently on endometriosis, so why not take that with you, and if you have any further questions please let me know.

Patient: Thank you very much for seeing me. Goodbye.

Doctor: Goodbye.

Explanations

1. **tummy:** abdomen.
2. **womb:** uterus.
3. **the pill:** contraceptive pill.
4. **put on:** increase.
5. **bloated:** distended.
6. **as long as:** provided.
7. **pass your motions:** defaecate.

8. **neck of the womb:** cervix.
9. **getting me down:** depressing me.
10. **works:** is effective.

29. Man, aged 74

Referred by his GP with a history of 3 months' increasing difficulty in walking with dragging of left leg. He had had several falls and was no longer able to get out of the house unaided.

Doctor: Good morning Mr York. Come and sit down. I'm Dr Butler. Your GP says you've had difficulty in getting about[1] for three months now and you can't go out alone. Would you like to tell me more about it?

Patient: Yes, that's right. My left leg seems to drag[2] behind. I can't walk properly at all. I just seem to shuffle[3] along so I daren't go out on my own.

Doctor: Your GP mentions you've fallen…

Patient: Yes, I've fallen several times in the house and cut my head open the last time.

Doctor: I'm sorry to hear that. Have you had any problems with your hands?

Patient: They've become very shaky. They've been like this for nearly a year but slowly getting worse. The left one is very bad.

Doctor: Is there anything else you've noticed?

Patient: Yes. I keep dribbling,[4] sometimes down my clothes. I'm embarrassed to see my old friends, I feel so awful. I used to try to keep up with[5] people by writing letters but now my hands are so trembly no-one can read my writing.

Doctor: Do you live alone then?

Patient: Yes. I lost[6] my wife three years ago with cancer. We'd been married forty years.

Doctor: Have you any children?

Patient: Yes, two daughters. One lives in Australia but the other lives half an hour away. She's very good and does my shopping for me.

Doctor: Has your GP organised any help from the Social Services for you?

Patient: She did get me meals on wheels[7] for a bit but I didn't like the food.

Doctor: You've had trouble with your stomach, have you?

Patient: Oh yes. I was in here with a perforated duodenal ulcer ten years ago. I have to be careful what I eat.

Doctor: Do you smoke?

Patient: Not now but I smoked thirty a day for twenty years. I suppose it takes its toll.[8]

Doctor: Have you had any other medical problems?

Patient: Well, I had a hernia operation fifteen years ago and my doctor said I had blood pressure so put me on tablets.

Doctor: What are they called do you know?

Patient: Yes, I've brought them to show you.

Doctor: Good. Bendrofluazide 2.5 mg daily. Well, Mr York I'd like to examine you now. Please go into the cubicle and take off your shoes and all your clothes except your pants and vest. Take your time. Would you like any help from the nurse?

Patient: No, I think I can manage.

Clinical notes

- Resting pillrolling tremor more in left arm
- Bradykinesia of fingers of both hands, more marked on left
- Cogwheel rigidity in left arm
- Reflexes normal
- Plantars downgoing
- Slightly shuffling gait
- Slightly stooped posture and flexed arms when walking
- CVS NAD

$$BP \frac{180}{90} \text{ lying}$$

$$\frac{180}{94} \text{ standing}$$

- RS NAD

- Abd. NAD
- Mini-mental state exam $\dfrac{27}{30}$ (i.e. no cognitive deficit)

Diagnosis

Parkinsonism probably due to idiopathic Parkinson's disease.

Doctor: Well, Mr York, I've had a good look at you and I'm pretty sure that all the problems you've been getting are due to Parkinson's disease.

Patient: Oh dear, that's serious, isn't it?

Doctor: It can be, but there's a lot we can do to help you. I'm going to give you some tablets called Sinemet. The tablets do occasionally make people slightly dizzy[9] on standing up or make them have vivid dreams or feel slightly muddled.[10] So I'll start you on a low dose (half a tablet twice daily) to try and avoid this. I'm also going to refer you to the physiotherapist to see how we can help you with your walking. Also I want you to see our occupational therapist who will assess you to see if you need any aids or adaptations to your house. This may involve a home visit. Is that clear?

Patient: Yes, thank you doctor.

Doctor: Good. Well I'll see you in a month's time to see how you are getting on.

Patient: Thank you very much.

Explanations

1. **getting about:** moving about, going out.
2. **drag:** move with difficulty, slowly.
3. **shuffle:** feet sliding, legs dragging, characteristic of Parkinsonism.
4. **dribble:** saliva flows from the mouth.
5. **keep up with:** keep in contact with.
6. **lost my wife:** my wife died.
7. **meals on wheels:** a service in which meals are taken to the homes of those in need such as invalids, the elderly.

8. **takes its toll:** causes illness.
9. **dizzy:** vertigo.
10. **muddled:** confused.

30. Man, aged 75

Had been living in Old Age Home for one year after death of his wife. Brought into hospital by his daughter and member of staff of Old Age Home.

Doctor: Hello Mr Harvey. How are you today?

Patient: I'm very upset. I want to go home.

Doctor: Well, let's see how you are and then we'll think about it. (to daughter) How long has he been in the Home?

Daughter: Since my mother died a year ago. Before that he was getting forgetful; couldn't remember what day it was, kept asking her the same questions over and over again. Nearly drove her mad. He often tripped over things so she was afraid to leave him alone in the end. When she died suddenly we tried to leave him in his own home because that's what he wanted. He lost nine pension books, and he just couldn't cope so he had to go into the Home.

Doctor: Do you live near him?

Daughter: No, we live fifty miles away. We both go out to work and have three children so it was out of the question for him to live with us.

Doctor: So how did you get on in the Home, Mr Harvey?

Patient: They told me I was going for two weeks and I've been there a year. The staff are dreadful, not helpful and nobody listens to me at all.

Doctor (to member of staff from Home): What were the problems?

Carer: He's very depressed, sleeps very badly and hardly eats. He's lost quite a bit of weight. Recently he's insulted quite a few people, started to be aggressive. Then two days ago he attacked one of the staff, tried to strangle her and scratched her arms and neck.

Doctor (to patient): Do you remember any of this happening?

Patient: No, of course not. It's not true. I would never act like that.

Doctor: Why are you here?

Patient: I don't know. I've no idea.

Doctor: Do you know where you are?

Patient: No. No. It's terrible. I just want to go home where I'm happy.

The patient is admitted to hospital and given simple memory tests and several simple tasks of reading, writing and drawing. Biochemical tests are taken. The results suggest Alzheimer's disease.

Doctor sees patient's daughter a week later:

Doctor: Hello, Mrs Cox, come and sit down. Well we've done a lot of tests and they show that your father probably has Alzheimer's disease. That accounts for his memory loss, his feelings of hopelessness and fits of aggression.

Daughter: Is there anything that can be done for him?

Doctor: Well, we can't do anything about his memory but we can help to change his mood and enjoy life more. We've got good new drugs which also slow down the memory deterioration. He should go back to the Old Age Home and try to enjoy some of the activities there. He can go to a Day Centre and perhaps make friends there.

Daughter: What's the long-term outlook?

Doctor: I can't say at this stage but we'll put him on the new tablets, check after two weeks to see how he's getting on. Our aim is for him to be as independent as possible. We would like to talk to you again after that.

Daughter: I'm most grateful for your help. Thank you.

Descriptive language of systems review

When a doctor has taken a history of the patient's complaints, it is customary to enquire whether the patient has complaints of any other system. Patients are not used to talking about their bodily functions and abnormalities and often cannot easily find the precise words to describe the character of pain, the consistency of stool, the tone of cough and so on.

Here are some of the questions that doctors ask repeatedly about urine, stools, sputum, etc. and the appropriate words to describe the colour, form and smell. It is difficult for a patient to be specific about the *amount* of blood, sputum and so on lost. A doctor, therefore, often suggests domestic utensils to give an idea of the measurement: 'How much sputum do you bring up? An egg-cupful?' Be sure you are familiar with the size of teaspoons, dessertspoons, tablespoons, egg-cup, tea-cup, etc.

BLOOD

— Blood; to bleed; bleeding.
— To lose blood; to have a haemorrhage; loss of blood.

Useful questions
— Have you had any loss of blood?
— Have you noticed any blood in your motions / in your sputum / when you pass water?
— Have you noticed any clots of blood?
— Was the blood bright or dark in colour?

Descriptive words
— Black; bright/dark; brown; coffee grounds; fresh/stale; heavy/

slight loss of blood; pink; watery; sticky; streaky with mucus.
— Arterial jetting.
— Capillary oozing.
— Venous flowing.

Colloquial expressions
— On the paper (as a result of haemorrhoids).
— Splash in the pan (blood from the rectum seen in the lavatory).
— Spotting (on the pants – intramenstrual bleeding).

BOWELS
— *Medical words:* faeces; stools; to defaecate.
— *Colloquial words:* motion or motions; to have the bowels opened. See pages 188–189 for examples of other colloquial expressions.

Useful questions
— How often do you have your bowels opened?
— Is this a life-long habit?
— What do the motions look like?
— Are they quite well formed?
— What about the colour? Has it changed?
— Are they darker in colour?
— Have you ever seen any blood in your motions?
— Have you noticed an unpleasant smell?
— Do you ever have diarrhoea or constipation?
— Do you have to go in a hurry?
— Can you hold your motions?
— Do you have to strain to pass your motions? (tenesmus)
— Do you take laxatives?
— Do the motions float on the water after flushing the lavatory?
— Do you ever have any pain on passing your motions?
— Do you get pain before, during or after passing your motions?
— Do you suffer from wind?
— Have you noticed any special food upsets your bowels?

— Have you lost any weight?

Descriptive words
— *Colour:* black; brown; burnt-looking; clay-like; colourless – like rice-water (cholera); dark brown; green; grey; pale; pea-soup-like; putty-like, porridge-like (steatorrhoea); redcurrant jelly-like; slatey grey; tarry; white; yellow.
— *Form and consistency:* bloody; bulky; crumbly; dry; fatty; floating; friable; frequent; frothy; greasy; hard; hard dry balls (scybalae); knobbly; large; loose; lumpy; pill-like; purulent (with pus); slimy (excess of mucus); soft; watery; well-formed; worms.
— *Amount:* copious; profuse; scanty.
— *Odour:* offensive – very bad smell.

BREATHING

— *Medical words:* respiration; expiration; inspiration.
— *Colloquial words:* breathing; breathing out; breathing in.

Useful questions
— Do you have any difficulty with your breathing?
— Is it more difficult to breathe in or breathe out?
— Do you get short of breath?
— Do you get short of breath when you run for a bus or climb stairs?
— Do you get any pain on breathing?
— Do you catch your breath?
— Do you gasp for air?
— Take a deep breath, hold your breath and then breathe out slowly.

Descriptive words
Breathless; deep; jerky; laboured; noisy; out of breath; puffed; quick; quiet; rapid; regular/irregular; shallow; shortness of breath; troubled; weak; wheezing.

CARDIOLOGY

Useful questions

— Do you ever have palpitations?

— If you have palpitations, how would you first become aware of them?

— Do they come on gradually or in some other way?

— Are there any other symptoms that you notice when you have palpitations?

— Are you ever aware of your heart beating fast?

— When your heart is beating fast can you tell whether it is beating regularly or irregularly?

— Do you have any chest discomfort or chest pain?

— Does the discomfort appear to be brought on by anything in particular?

— Does the chest discomfort, for instance, occur more commonly when you are sitting in a chair or when you are walking?

— When you have your chest discomfort/pain, have you noticed that it is accompanied by anything else?

— What do you do when you get your chest pain (or chest discomfort)?

— Does position make any difference to your chest discomfort/pain?

— Do you ever get chest discomfort/pain at night?

— If you take the trinitrin (or tablet under the tongue) how quickly does this help relieve the chest discomfort/pain?

— Does the chest discomfort/pain spread anywhere else in the body?

— Do you ever become dizzy?

— Have you ever fainted?

— Before you actually faint, are you aware that you are about to faint?

— If you have a fainting episode can you describe the sequence of events leading up to it?

— Do you actually lose consciousness or are you aware of your surroundings and people talking?

— Do you actually fall to the ground?
— When you feel faint, are you able to steady yourself against the wall or an object?
— Do you sometimes feel faint when you get up from a chair or out of a hot bath?
— Could you try beating out the rate and the rhythm for me with your hand?
— How long have your ankles been swollen?
— Are they swollen first thing in the morning?
— How far can you walk?
— Can you walk as far as you could five years ago?
— How many steps can you climb?

COUGH

Useful questions
— How long have you had a cough?
— Did anything special bring it on?
— What kind of cough is it?
— When do you get it?
— Does any position make it worse?
— Do you bring anything up?
— Do you get a pain in your chest when you cough?

Descriptive words
— *Tone:* barking; brassy; hacking; hawking (catarrhal and chronic sinusitis); husky; staccato; stridulous; wheezing (bronchitis).
— *Character:* dry/productive, explosive/suppressed; postural / not postural; spasmodic/persistent, choking; painful; smoker's cough (means coughing early morning); tickling; tight.

DISCHARGE

— A discharge.
— To discharge.

Useful questions

— How long have you had this discharge from your ear/eyes /nose/rectum/vagina?
— How often do you get it?
— How much is there?
— What colour is it?
— Does it contain casts, clots, mucus, pus?

Descriptive words

— *Colour:* brownish-yellow; creamy-white; green; yellow.
— *Type:* blood-stained; frothy; itchy; jelly-like; milky; with pus; with serum.
— *Odour:* foetid; foul-smelling; offensive.

LOCOMOTOR

Useful questions

— Do you have any pain or stiffness in any joints?
— Do you have any pain or stiffness in your limbs, your neck or back?
— How long does the stiffness last?
— Do you have any tingling in the hands or feet?
— Is it worse in the morning or evening?
— Any swelling?
— Are there any movements that you now find difficult?
— Does it affect your daily living?
— Have you had a skin rash?
— Have you noticed a discharge down below?
— Have you had any ulcers in your mouth?
— Have you noticed any dryness of your mouth or eyes?
— If you go out into the cold, do your fingers change colour and become painful?

MENSTRUATION

— To menstruate: to have one's period(s).

— See page 189 for examples of other colloquial expressions.

Useful questions
— When did your periods first start?
— How often do you get/have/see your periods?
— How long do they last?
— How much do you lose? Are they heavy?
— If patient replies 'Yes':
— How many pads do you use each day?
— Do you wear pads as well as tampons?
— Do you ever pass clots? How big are they?
— Do you get pain before or during your periods?
— How do you feel before your periods start?
— Do you feel edgy (nervous) irritable?
— Do you get any bleeding after intercourse or between your periods?
— When was your last period?

The menopause
— See page 198 for examples of colloquial expressions.
— Are you still having your periods?
— Are they regular?
— When did you see the last one?
— Do you get hot flushes and sweats? How often?
— Do the flushes interrupt your sleep?
— Do you have any trouble when you have intercourse?
— Do you have soreness or dryness?
— Do you have bleeding after intercourse?
— Do you have itching?
— Have you had any bleeding since your periods stopped?
— Have you had any discharge?

NEUROLOGY

Useful questions
— Do you suffer from headaches?

— Are they worse in the morning or evening?
— In which part of the head do you get the pain?
— Do you ever feel sick or vomit?
— Does the light hurt your eyes?
— Any other trouble with your eyes?
— Have you noticed any blurring of vision?
— Do you ever see things double?
— Do you ever see flashing lights?
— Have you had any fits, faints or funny turns?
— Was there any warning you were going to have a fit?
— Did you bite your tongue?
— Did you wet yourself?
— Do you have any problems with your hearing?
— Have you noticed any numbness, tingling or weakness in your limbs?
— Are you passing more water than you used to?
— Can you control your bowel movements?

OBSTETRICS

— To be pregnant: to be expecting a baby.
— See pages 189, 190, 198 and 199 for examples of other colloquial expressions.

Useful questions

— Is this your first pregnancy?
— How many children have you?
— How old are they?
— How long did your pregnancy last?
— Did you have any trouble during pregnancy such as raised blood pressure?
— Was labour induced or did it start by itself?
— How long were you in labour?
— Did you have a normal delivery/forceps/Caesarian operation?
— Have you had any miscarriages (spontaneous abortions)?
— At what stage of pregnancy were they?

PAIN

Pain and ache mean the same thing and we speak of 'aches and pains' generally. Both these words are nouns but the word 'ache' can be used with the following to form a compound noun: backache; earache; headache; stomach-ache; toothache. For the other parts of the body we say, 'I have a pain in my shoulder', chest, etc.

It is possible to have a pain in the back, head and stomach but this generally refers to a more serious condition than backache, headache and stomach-ache.

The word 'ache' can also be used as a verb: 'My leg aches after walking ten miles' or 'My back aches after gardening'.

The word 'hurt' is another verb used to express injury and pain: 'My chest hurts when I cough' or 'My neck hurts when I turn my head'.

Useful questions

— *Duration:* How long have you had this pain?
— *Site:* Where do you get the pain? Show me exactly where you get the pain.
— *Character:* What kind of pain is it?
— *Onset:* Did it come on slowly or suddenly?
— *Time:* When do you get the pain?
— *Severity:* Does it wake you up at night?
— *Cause:* Does anything special bring it on? (emotional disturbance, exercise, food, position, etc).
  Does anything special make it worse?
— *Radiation:* Does it spread anywhere else?
— *Relief:* Does anything relieve it? (drug, exercise, food, heat, position, rest).
— *Character:* The type of pain is important in differential diagnosis. You do not want to suggest the character but if the patient is vague in answering 'What kind of pain is it?' then you must offer one or two suitable words such as 'Is it a throbbing or a cutting pain?'. The following are the most commonly used words to describe pain:

- beating;
- biting;
- boring;
- burning, (as in cystitis, ulcer);
- bursting;
- colicky (abdominal disease);
- crampy;
- cutting (rectal disease);
- dragging;
- drawing;
- dull (headache, tumour);
- gnawing (tumour), pronounced gnawing;
- grinding;
- griping;
- gripping (as in angina pectoris);
- heavy (as pre-menstrual);
- knife-like;
- numb (lack of sensation);
- piercing (angina pectoris);
- pinching;
- pounding (headache)
- pressing;
- prickling (like pins and needles in inflamed eyes, conjunctivitis);
- scalding (cystitis);
- severe pain — gip, 'It gives me the gip';
- sharp;
- shooting (sciatica, toothache);
- sickening;
- smarting (burns);
- sore;
- spiky
- splinter-like
- stabbing (indigestion);
- stinging (cuts, stings);
- stitch (spasm in side due to excessive exercise);

- straining;
- tearing;
- tender;
- throbbing (headache);
- tingling (return of circulation to extremities);
- twinge (sudden, sharp).
- twisting
— *Other words to describe pain:* acute; agonising; chronic; constant; constricting; convulsive; darting; deep-seated; difficult to move; diffuse; excruciating; fleeting; intense; intermittent; localised; mild; obstinate; persistent; radiating; severe; spasmodic; spreading; stubborn; superficial; very severe; violent.

PSYCHIATRY

Useful questions
— How has your mood been lately?
— Have you felt sad or depressed?
— Have you felt like crying at all?
— Have you felt anxious or worried?
— Have you felt frightened about anything?
— Are you finding it difficult to cope with life at the moment?
— Do you get angry more easily than usual?
— How've you been sleeping?
— Do you have any difficulty falling asleep?
— Do you wake up earlier than usual?
— Are you eating normally?
— Do you have a good appetite?
— Are you losing weight?
— Are you able to enjoy the things you normally do?
— Have you lost interest in things around you?
— How do you see the future turning out?
— Do you think it's possible for you to get better?
— Do you ever feel life isn't worth living any more?
— Do you ever think about wanting to die or wishing you were dead?

— Do you ever have any thoughts about harming yourself?
— Do you ever feel yourself sweating more than usual?
— Do you ever feel your heart pounding?
— Does your mouth go dry?
— Is there anything particular that brings these feelings on?
— When you feel tense and anxious, is there anything that makes you feel better?
— Have you had any trouble with your nerves?
— Do you live with anyone?
— Have you anyone you can talk to about your problems?
— How long have you been in the same job?
— Do you enjoy your work?

Drinking habits
(See p. 191 for examples of colloquial expressions.)
— Do you drink at all?
— Do you drink every day or just on social occasions?
— Roughly, how much do you drink on average every day?
— Do you drink alone?
— Do you drink in the mornings?
— Have you ever been a drinker?
— Do you ever feel guilty about your drinking?
— Have you ever tried to cut down your drinking?
— Have you ever had any fits or black-outs through drinking?
— Do you think your drinking causes any problems? At work? With your marriage? With relationships with other people?
— Have you ever got into trouble with the law through drinking?

PULSE

Useful question
— Do you get palpitations? (See Cardiology, p. 170)

Descriptive words
Absent; bounding; collapsing; faint; fast; feeble; frequent; full; gal-

loping; hard; intermittent; irregular (a) regularly irregular (extrasystole), (b) irregularly irregular (atrial fibrillation); jerking; low; quick; rapid; regular; slow; small; soft; strong; tensed; thready; vibrating; weak.

SKIN

Useful questions
— Do you have any problems with your skin?
— Have you ever had a skin rash?
— Any itching of the skin?
— Do you have any allergies?
— Is there eczema or psoriasis in your family?
— What medication are you using?
— Are you using anything on your skin?

SPUTUM

— *Medical words:* sputum; to expectorate.
— *Colloquial words:* phlegm (pronounced flem); to bring up phlegm; spit.

Useful questions
— Do you bring up any phlegm?
— How much do you bring up?
— When do you bring it up?
— What colour is it?
— Have you noticed any blood?
— Is it frothy, watery, etc?
— Is there a lot of blood or just streaky with blood?

Descriptive words
— *Colour:* black-grey; blood-flecked; blood-stained; bright red; brown; dark red; green; pinkish; prune juice-like; raspberry-like; rusty-brown (pneumonia); streaked; yellow.

— *Quality:* clear; frothy; glassy; jelly-like; opaque; presence of cysts, bile, pellets, etc.; sticky; thick; thin; transparent.
— *Odour:* foetid; nauseating; putrid.

UROLOGY

— *Medical words:* to micturate; to urinate.
— *Colloquial words:* to pass water. See page 190 for examples of other colloquial expressions.

Useful questions
— Do you have any difficulty in passing your water?
— Is the difficulty when you start passing your water, throughout or afterwards?
— Does your water gush?
— Does your water dribble?
— Does it come away when you cough, laugh, sneeze or strain?
— How often do you pass water?
— Do you have to get up in the night (to pass water)?
— Has the amount of water you pass increased/decreased?
— How much urine do you pass each time?
— Have you noticed any change in the colour of your water?
— Have you seen any blood in your water?
— Have you noticed an unusual smell?
— Do you have any pain when you pass your water?
— Does your water burn or sting?
— I'd like to have a specimen (sample) of your water.
— I'd like to have a mid-stream specimen.

Descriptive words
— *Colour:* amber; black; brown; blood-streaked; blue-green (as result of drugs for back and kidney); bright red; dark brown; orange; pink; red; reddish-brown; straw-coloured (normal); yellow.
— *Character:* clear; cloudy; flecked; foaming; frothy; milky; muddy; thick; transparent; turbid; slimy; smoky.
— *Odour:* ammoniacal; fishy; foetid; fruity and sweet (diabetes).

VOMITING

— *Medical word:* to vomit.
— *Colloquial words:* to be sick; to bring up food. Note: nausea; colloquial expression is to feel sick. See page 190–191 for examples of other colloquial expressions.

Useful questions

— When were you sick? (this means: When did you vomit?)
— Do you feel better after being sick (or after vomiting)?
— How often do you vomit?
— How much do you vomit?
— What colour is the vomit?
— Have you noticed any coffee grounds, bile, blood in your vomit?
— When do you vomit?
— Is it related to eating?
— Do you feel sick before you vomit or does it just happen?
— Do you retch?

Descriptive words

— *Colour:* black; blood; coffee-grounds; green.
— *Character:* copious; frothy; residues of food; watery fluid.
— *Odour:* Sour-smelling.

SENTENCES FOR ALL PARTS OF THE BODY

These sentences cover most parts of the body that your patient will speak of. Most of the sentences come from case histories, others are from medical reports. Notice the structure of the sentence and the use of tenses. From these sentences you can make dozens more by simply changing the details. Look at these examples:

— I've had this ➤ *swelling* on my ➤ *neck* for ➤ *two weeks.*
  lump   *breast*   *six weeks.*
  spot   *eyelid*   *three months.*
  ulcer   *tongue*   *five days.*

— When I'm tired, ➤ *my eyelid flickers.*
    my head aches.
    my back aches.
    I can't sleep properly.
    I can't eat.

By developing this method, you will be sure of making a perfect English sentence. It will also help you to stop translating from your own language.

HEAD AND NECK

— The man suffered from recurring intense *headaches*.
— My *hair* has been dropping out for the past three months.
— Since I had shingles, I've had a deadness and a tingling feeling in my *forehead*.
— I keep getting a sharp pain in my *temple*.
— When I'm tired, my *eyelid* flickers.
— *Her eyelashes* have grown in the wrong direction. They rub on the *cornea* and cause irritation.
— When a patient is jaundiced, *the whites of his eyes* are yellow.
— I have a strange creepy feeling on my *scalp*.
— The patient had felt generally unwell for some time and then she noticed she had pink spots all over her *face*.
— The boy's *pupils* were dilated as a result of drugs.
— There is some hard wax in this *ear*. I'll give you some drops to soften it.
— I've got terrible catarrh and can't breathe through my *nose*.
— I've found I have a lump inside my *mouth* and I'm worried about it.
— In winter my *lips* are cracked.
— I'm afraid you'll have to have this *tooth* extracted.
— When I brush my *teeth*, my *gums* bleed.
— In undulant fever (brucellosis, Malta Fever) the *tongue* frequently has a central white fur.
— You've come out in a rash all over your *cheek*.

— The child fell down and cut open his *chin*. He had to have five stitches in it.

— In tetanus, stiffness of the *jaw* occurs until the patient is unable to open his *mouth*.

— I've had this swelling on my *neck* for two weeks.

— When I eat, I can't swallow properly. It feels as if everything is sticking in my *throat*.

ARMS AND HANDS

— The old woman slipped and dislocated her *shoulder*.

— I've had pain and swelling under my *arm* (in my *armpit*) for several weeks.

— When I play tennis, I get a pain in my *elbow* and it is painful to straighten my *arm*.

— Last year I broke my *arm* and had to have it in plaster.

— When he was playing cricket, he sprained his *wrist*. It was painful and swollen.

— The man who worked with a pneumatic drill said in winter his *hands* were numb and painful.

— The girl noticed irritation on the *palm of her hand* and between the *fingers* and it turned out to be scabies.

— I was washing the floor and a pin went into my *thumb*. Half of it is broken inside.

— My *knuckles* are so swollen when I wake up.

— The old man was unable to clench his *fist*.

— My *nails* keep on breaking and splitting.

LEGS AND FEET

— The man's *leg* was amputated because gangrene set in.

— I'm going into hospital next week to have these veins on my *thighs* stripped.

— I keep getting a lot of pain in my left *knee*. Sometimes it feels as if it will give way.

— The man had severe pain in his *calves* when he was walking. After a short rest the pain went off.

— She was walking along when suddenly she felt a severe pain in her *foot*.

— The boy sprained his *ankle* playing football. It became blue, swollen and painful.

— She had trouble with her *feet*. They were covered with chilblains in winter and she had a bunion on her *big toe* and a *hammer toe*.

— My little boy gets swelling and tenderness at the back of his *heel* and it is so painful that he limps.

BODY

— I keep getting a stabbing pain in my *chest* and I get out of breath when I go upstairs.

— Many women have pain and fullness in their *breasts* before their period.

— One of the signs of cancer of the breast is *nipple* retraction.

— A 34-year-old woman had been found to have a *heart* murmur during her first pregnancy six years previously.

— I get a sharp pain in my *side* when I crouch or stand up.

— The man fell from a ladder and broke two of his *ribs*.

— I've got arthritis in my *hip* and some days I can hardly move.

— I get a burning pain and a blown-up feeling in my *stomach*.

— I mustn't eat rich food because I've had *gallstones* for years.

— I've noticed blood in my motions and I get a pain in my *back passage* (anus).

— I'm having a lot of trouble with my *bowels*. Sometimes I'm constipated and then I get diarrhoea.

— She has had *bladder* trouble since she was a child.

— I'm afraid we shall have to remove the *womb*.

— The patient complained of a swelling in the *groin* and a *vaginal* discharge.

— I keep wanting to pass water and I have a pain in my *back*. Do you think it's *kidney* trouble, doctor?

— I've got a pain in my *private parts* (penis).

Colloquial English

7

LANGUAGE USED BY PATIENTS TO DISCUSS SYMPTOMS

Many patients, especially the elderly, find extreme difficulty in discussing their bodily functions and symptoms of disorder with a doctor. This may be from ignorance or shyness. Obviously the more intimate the part of the body, the greater the embarrassment, and so a wide vocabulary of euphemisms and slang expressions has sprung up in the English language. Some of them are used by uneducated people, others by embarrassed educated people.

Quite often the patient is so inarticulate that the doctor has to suggest various symptoms and the patient merely says 'yes' or 'no'. In this case, the doctor often uses colloquial expressions himself which he thinks the patient will understand.

Regional expressions have been mainly excluded in the following chapters. Those phrases which are most commonly used have been printed in italics, for example, *back passage*. Those which are not commonly used in polite society, have been marked with an asterisk,*.

PARTS OF THE BODY

Anus – arse*, arsehole*, *back passage*, butt*, butthole*, hole*.
To break wind: to fart*, to poop*, to trump*.
Bladder – waterworks, e.g. Doctor to patient: 'How are the waterworks?'
How is your bladder working?
Bowels – gut, e.g. a pain in one's gut, to have belly ache (often used to mean bowels), to have gut ache.

Brain – head-piece.

Breast – boobs*, *bosom*, buffers*, charleys*, *chest*, chestnut*, globe*, knockers*, nipples, paps*, tits*, titties*, top part. Imitation breasts: falsies. Small breasts: 'I haven't got much'.

Buttocks – arse*, backside, *behind, bottom*, botty (childish), bum*, buns* (male), cheeks, hind quarters, posterior, rear, rump*, *seat, sit-me-down* (nursery), sit-upon, stern, tail, toby. To have large buttocks: to be broad in the beam.

Cervix – neck of womb.

Chest – to have a *flat*, barrel, *hollow*, pigeon chest.
  The following are only used for females:
      bosom, breast, buffers*, *bust*.
  To have a bad cough: *to bark*.
  Coughing: *to be chesty, a bit chesty*.
  To have one's chest finger-tapped: to have a thump.

Clitoris – clit*.

Crotch – often used to mean groin or skin covering genitalia.

Ear – 'bat ears (prominent), a cauliflower ear (from boxing), flappers, lug*, (e.g. to have lugache*).
  Rather deaf: to be hard of hearing.

Elbow – *funny bone*, e.g. *to hit one's funny bone* (so called because of the strange tingling one experiences when it is struck).

Eyes – glimmers*, ogles*, optics, peepers.
  To have a squint: to be boss-eyed, to be cock-eyed, to be wall-eyed.
  To have low visual acuity in one eye: to have a lazy eye.

Face – clock*, dial*, mug*, physog*.

Genitals – male and female: bits, package, *down below, private parts*, thing, pencil and tassle* (male child's penis and scrotum), twig and berries* (male child's penis and testicles).

Hand – mitt, paw.

Head – bonce; brain-box, brain-pan, napper, nob, noddle, nous-box (nous means intelligence, common sense), nut, *skull*.

Heart – engine, e.g. 'my engine's not working properly', jam tart* (Cockney), *ticker*.

Something wrong with one's heart: to have a cardiac heart, *to have a dicky heart.*

To have a weak heart: to have a heart.

Hymen – maidenhead, maid's ring (Cockney).

Intestines – bowels, guts, innards, *inside.*

Legs – bandy legged (bow), drumsticks (very thin), K-legged (with knees knocking together), knock-kneed (knees bent inwards to face each other), peg leg (a wooden leg), pins, spindles.

A lame leg: to have a gammy leg.

Short legs: to have duck's disease.

Walk badly: to be bad on one's pins.

Walking with the feet turned in: hen-toed.

Lungs – bellows, tubes.

To be bad in one's breathing: *to be short-winded.*

Mouth – chops*, gob* trap*.

Navel – belly button.

Neck – Adam's apple (projection of thyroid cartilage of larynx), salt cellars (very deep hollows above collar-bone in female neck), scruff of neck (nape).

Nose – beacon* (red and large), beak*, conk*, hooter*, sniffer*, snitch*.

Nasal congestion: to be blocked up, bunged up, *stuffy.*

Nasal discharge: snot*.

Noisy breathing in children due to nasal congestion: snuffles.

Running nose: a snotty nose*.

Penis – almond*, almond rock* (Cockney), bean*, button* (baby), club*, cock*, dick*, equipment*, gear*, it*, John Thomas*, knob*, little man*, little tail* (small boys), meat*, old man*, Peter*, pinkle*, prick*, *private parts, privates,* rod*, shaft*, she*, stick*, tadger* (Northern England), tassel*, thing*, tool*, Will*, Willie*.

Scrotum – bag*.

Skull – brain pan.

Spine – backbone.

Stomach – abdomen, belly, bread-basket*, corporation (when large), croop, guts (stomach and intestines), innards, inner man, peenie, pinafore, *tummy*.

To belch: *to burp*.

The noise the stomach makes when one is hungry: *to have stomach rumbles*.

Something wrong with it: to have a gastric stomach.

Stomach ache: to have a pain in one's guts.

Distension of stomach in older people – middle age spread.

Teeth – buck teeth (protruding); peggy, peggies (nursery talk).

Testicles – ballocks*, balls*, bollocks*, charleys*, cobblers*, cods*, nuts*, pills*, pillocks*, stones*. See **Genitals.**

Throat – clack*, gullet, organ-pipe (wind-pipe).

A very severe cough: a churchyard cough.

Sputum: *phlegm*.

To be hoarse: *to have a frog in the throat*.

To have a sore throat: to have a throat.

Tongue – clack*, clapper*.

The tongue can be described as: coated, dirty, *furred*, furry, thick.

Talkative person: *a chatterbox*.

Trachea – *windpipe*.

Urethra – pipe.

Vagina (or vulva) – birth canal, box*, brush*, crack*, cunt*, *down below*, fanny*, *front passage*, hair pie*, it, private, e.g. 'my private is sore', *private part*, pubes*, pussy*, slit*, thing*, there, twat*, up inside.

Umbilicus – *navel*.

Uterus – box, *womb*.

BODILY FUNCTIONS

Defaecate, to – to crap*, to do a big job, to do a job, to do a pooh (childish), to do a rear*, to do number two, to do one's business, to go to the toilet (and use paper), to have a clear out, *to have the bowels opened*, to job*, *to pass one's motions*, to shit*, *to use a bedpan* (hospital).

Faeces, stools – baby's yellow (infantile excrement), business, cack*, job*, mess*, *motions*, number two, shit*.

Doctor to patient: 'Are your motions well formed?'.

Mothers often say of a child: 'His toilet is green' (meaning his stools are green).

Note that 'a dose of salts' means Epsom salts.

Tenesmus: *straining.*

Constipation, to have – to be costive, *I haven't been for four days.* I haven't had a road through me for a week*.

Diarrhoea, to have – back door trots*, collywobbles, Gippy tummy, run'ems, runs, scours, squitters.

To have a sudden attack of diarrhoea: *to be taken short.*

Die, to – to be a goner, to be all over, to be slipping (to be dying), to burn oneself out (die early through overwork), to conk out, to go (go away), to go home, to go to the next world, to hang up one's hat, to have had it, to have one's number up, to have had one's chips, to have one foot in the grave (to be dying), to kick the bucket, *to pass away*, to peg out, to pip out, to pop off (usually die suddenly), to push up daisies, to snuff it or out, to turn it in, to turn one's toes up, *to have had a long* (or *good*) *innings* (to die at an old age), *to lay out* (prepare for burial).

Note: to commit suicide: to kill oneself.

Faint, to – *to black out, to have a black-out,* to go off hooks, to pass out.

Impotent, to become – to be no good to one's wife, to lose one's nature.

A man's impotence will be expressed by his wife in the following ways: he can't sustain an erection, *he can't manage*, his cock's soft or droopy*.

Menstruate, to – to be unwell, *one's period, the curse,* the days, the monthlies, the other, the thing, *the time of the month,* the usual.

'Have you seen anything?' (feminine euphemism).

'I haven't seen for six weeks' (no menstruation, probably pregnant).

Doctor to patient: 'When was your last period?'

Naked, to be – to be in one's birthday suit, to be in the altogether, to be starkers.

Pregnant, to be – away the trip* (Scottish working class), to be caught*, *to be expecting, to be having a baby*, to be in a delicate condition, to be in an interesting condition, to be in Kittle (Scottish), to be in pig*, to be in pod*, to be in the club*, to be in the family way, to be in the pudding club*, to be one in line*, to be preggers*, to be up the pole*, to be up the stick*, to catch on, to catch the virus*, to click*, to cop it*, to fall for a baby (to have an unwanted pregnancy), to have a bun in the oven*, to have a touch of the sun*.

She's six months pregnant: she's six months gone. (See pages 198–199 for further examples.)

Fluttering sensation felt by woman when pregnant: quickening.

Sleep, to – to close one's eyes, *to doze* (short sleep), to go off (to fall asleep), to go to the land of nod, *to have a cat-nap* (short sleep), *to have a doze, to have a snooze* (short sleep), *to have forty winks* (short sleep), *to have some shut-eye, to nod off* (short sleep), ziz.

Urinate, to (micturate) – to do number one, *to go to the loo*, to have a run-out, *to pass water*, to pee, to pee-wee (childish), to piddle*, to piss*, *to spend a penny* (women only), to tiddle (childish), to tinkle (women only), to wee-wee (childish).

Nocturia: to get up in the night.

Hostess to guests: 'Do you want to wash your hands?' (do you want to go to the toilet?).

The lavatory can be described as: *bathroom*, bog*, *cloakroom*, convenience, *Gents'*, heads*, *Ladies'*, lav., lavvy, little girls' room, *loo*, place, powder room (Ladies' in a hotel), privies, rears*, *toilet*, WC.

A chamber pot: banjo*, gerry*, po, pot, potty (childish).

To hold a baby over a chamber pot: to hold out a baby.

To put a baby on a chamber pot: to pot.

Vomit, to – to be ill, *to be sick*, to bring up, to lose the lot, to puke*, to pump your heart up, to sick up, to spew*, to throw up*.

Nausea: the sicks.

To have nausea: to feel queasy, *to feel sick*.

'Have you vomited?' '*Have you been sick?*'.

To try to vomit but nothing comes up: *to retch*.

To vomit very much: to be as sick as a dog (or cat).

To have a headache and vomiting: to have a sick headache.

Weep, to – to blub, to blubber, to break down, *to cry*, to turn on the waterworks, to turn the tap on.

MENTAL AND PHYSICAL STATES

Angry, to be – to be cross, to be crusty, to be heated, to be hot under the collar, to be liverish, to be livid, to be shirty, to be steamed up, to flip, to fly off the handle, to go off the deep end, to have a paddy, to have a tantrum, to jump down someone's throat, to let off steam, to lose one's hair, to lose one's shirt, to play the devil, to see red.

Depressed, to be – to be blue, to be browned-off, to be down in the hips, to be down in the mouth, to be fed up, to be in the dumps, to be low, to be off the hinges, to have a button on, to have a chopper, to have a face as long as a fiddle, to have the droops, to have the hump, to have the hyp, to have the mopes, to have the pip.

Drunk, to be – to be a dipso (dipsomaniac), to be boozed (boozy), to be fou*, to be fresh (slightly drunk), to be fuddled (confused with drink), to be high, to be high on surge (to be drunk on surgical spirit), to be lush (slightly drunk), to be merry (happy with drink), to be muzzed, to be on the bottle (habitual drinker), to be paralytic (very drunk), to be plastered, to be slewed, to be sloshed, to be soaked (very drunk), to be sozzled (very drunk), to be squiffy (slightly drunk), to be stoned (very drunk), to be tiddly (slightly drunk), to be tight, to be tipsy (slightly drunk), to be under the influence (of liquor), to be well-oiled, to be woozy (confused with drink), to have a skinful (very drunk), to have Dutch courage (extra courage induced by drink), to have more than one can carry, to have one over the eight, to see pink elephants (or spiders) (to suffer from DTs), to have a hang-over (to feel ill as a result of drink), to have a morning-after-the-night-before (to feel ill as a result of drink), to hit the bottle (to drink excessively).

Dull, to be – to be a dream, a drip, a moron, a muggins, a noodle, a pie-can, a sap*, a wet, dead alive, dopey, dumb, foolish, goofy, half-baked, half-witted, lethargic, mutton-headed, silly, simple, slack, slow, soft, stupid, thick, thick-skulled.

Exhausted, to be – to be all in, to be clapped out*, to be dead, to be done for, done in, done up, to be fagged out, to be finished, to be flaked out, to be jiggered, to be knackered*, to be knocked up, to be ready to drop, to be shagged*, to be shattered, *to be tired out*, to be used up (utterly exhausted), *to be weary*, to be whacked, to feel like death, to go all to pieces (collapse from exhaustion).

To knock it out of one, '*walking uphill knocks it out of me*' (walking uphill exhausts me).

Healthy, to be – to be A1, to be as fit as a box of birds, to be as fit as a fiddle, to be fighting fit, to be first rate, to be full of beans, to be in fine fettle, to be in the pink, to be on good form, to have plenty of pep (pep = energy), to have plenty of vim (energy, vigour), to perk up (recover good health).

To begin to recover after an illness: *to be on the mend*, to turn the corner.

Madness – (in varying degrees): to be a bit touched, to be a case, to be a character (to be eccentric, odd), a scatterbrain (very forgetful, vague), to be as mad as a hatter, balmy, (barmy), batty, bats, bonkers, to be clean gone, cracked, crackers, crack-pot, crank, crazy, to be dippy, dotty, gaga (senile decay), goofy, half-baked, kinky, loony, loopy, mad, to be MD (mentally deficient), to be mental, non compos mentis, not all there, to be not right in one's head, nuts, off one's block, off one's chump, off one's head, off one's nut, off one's rocker, to be off the rails, out of one's mind, to be peculiar, potty, round the bend, scatty, screwy, a screwball, silly, simple, soft, stupid, up the creek, weak in the upper storey, to go doolally, to go hay-wire, to have bats in the belfry, with a tile (or screw) missing (or loose).

Mental hospital: bin, funny farm, loony bin, nuthouse.

To threaten to lock someone up as a madman: to put in a strait jacket.

Nervous, to feel – to be a fuss-pot, to be a jitter-bug, to be all hot and bothered, to be all of a dither, to be chewed up, *to be edgy*, on edge, to be fidgety, to be in a blue funk, to be in a flap, to be in a stew, to be in a tizzy, to be jittery, to be screwed up, to be shook-up (nerve-racked), to get all het-up, *to get in a state*, to get uptight, to go all hot and cold, to go into a flat spin, to go to pieces (collapse through nerves), to go up the wall, to have ants in one's pants*, to have butterflies in one's stomach, to have forty fits, to have kittens, to have the creeps, to have the heebie-jeebies, to have the shakes, to have the shivers, to have the twitters, to have the willies, to have the wind up, to have the worrits, to lose one's cool, to worrit (be anxious).

Unwell, to be – to be anyhow, to be below par, to be C_3 (very unfit), to be groggy, to be not oneself, to be not quite right, *to be off colour*, to be out of sorts, to be peaky, to be pingley, to be poorly, *to be run down*, to be taken bad, to be tenpence to the bob, *to be under the weather*, to be washed-out, to be weedy (anaemic, sickly), to be wobbly (weak after an illness), to be wonky (weak), to come all over queer, faint, ill (suddenly feel unwell), to crack up, to feel a bit off it, to feel a bit rough, to feel funny, to feel half-baked, to feel like death warmed up (very unwell), to feel like nothing on earth, to feel lousy, to feel queer, to feel ragged, to feel seedy, to go funny, to have a bad turn.

Vertigo – *to be dizzy*, to be giddy, to be muzzy, to feel the room spin, to feel queer, to have a mazy bout, to have a swimming head.

DISEASES AND OTHER CONDITIONS

Medical name	*Colloquial name*
Alopecia	baldness
Angina pectoris	angina

Arteriosclerosis	hardening of the arteries
Blepharitis	stye
Brucellosis	undulant fever
Bursitis	housemaid's knee
Cancer	a growth
Candida	thrush
Cerebral concussion	to be concussed, to be knocked out
Cerebral palsy	to be spastic
Cerebral embolism, haemorrhage or thrombosis	apoplexy, seizure, stroke
Chorea	St Vitus' dance
Colic	gripes
Conjunctivitis	pink eye
Contusion	bruise
Convulsions	fits
Coronary thrombosis; myocardial infarction	a coronary, heart attack
Coryza	cold in the head
Dandruff	scurf
Delirium tremens	DTs, the jerks, the shakes
Diabetes mellitus	sugar
Dysmenorrhoea	painful periods
Dysphagia	difficulty swallowing
Dyspnoea	breathless, out of breath, puffed, short of breath
Dyspepsia	indigestion
Encephalitis	brain fever
Encephalitis lethargica	sleepy sickness
Enuresis	bed-wetting
Epilepsy	fits, the shakes
Epistaxis	nosebleeds
Eructation	belching
Erythema pernio	chilblains
Flatulence, flatus	wind, Note: to belch (to send

	out wind from stomach noisily), to fart* (to send out wind from anus)
Frequency	I keep wanting to go (to pass urine)
Furuncle	boil
Gonorrhea	clap
Haemorrhoids	piles
Halitosis	bad breath
Hernia	rupture
Herpes simplex	cold blister or sore
Herpes zoster	shingles
Hordeolum	stye
Hydrops	dropsy
Hydrophobia	rabies
Hypertension	high blood pressure
Incontinence	leaky, not to be able to hold one's water or motions, to have an accident
Infectious mononucleosis	glandular fever
Infective hepatitis	catarrhal jaundice
Influenza	'flu
Leucorrhoea	whites
Luxation	dislocation, to put out a joint
Lymphadenoma	Hodgkin's disease
Menopause	the change (of life); the turn (of life)
Menstruation	period(s)
Monilia	thrush
Myopia	short-sight
Nephritis	Bright's disease
Neuralgia	face ache
Nocturia	to get up at night (to pass water)
Oedema	dropsy, swelling
Osteoporosis	brittle bone disease

Parotitis (viral)	mumps
Peritonsillar abscess	quinsy
Pertussis	whooping cough
Poliomyelitis	infantile paralysis; polio
Pruritus	itching
Pyrexia	fever, a temperature
Pyrosis	heartburn, water-brash
Raynaud's disease	white or dead fingers
Recurrent appendicitis	grumbling appendix
Rheumatism	screws, springes, rheumatics
Rubella	German measles
Rubeola; morbilli	measles
Scabies	the itch
Scarlatina	scarlet fever
Strabismus	squinting
Syncope	fainting
Tachycardia	palpitations
Tendonitis	golfer's elbow, tennis elbow
Tetanus	lockjaw
Tinea circinata	ringworm
Tinnitus	ringing in the ears
Tuberculosis	consumption; TB
Urticaria	hives, heat spots; nettle rash
Varicella	chickenpox
Variola	smallpox
Verrucae	warts
Venous thrombosis	white leg (in pregnancy)
Vesicle	blister

MEDICINE

(*In this section the text in bold type is the colloquial expression*)

Capsules – unpleasant drugs contained in a soluble case.

Dope, physic – any kind of medicine.

Medicine – anything taken to relieve pain or symptoms of illness. Usually the word refers to liquid or drugs taken by mouth.

Pills, tablets – drugs in tablet form. Note: to be on the pill: to be taking the contraceptive pill.

A tonic – medicine to invigorate one after an illness.

To be at death's door, to be critical, to be nearly a goner – to be dangerously ill.

To be laid up – to be confined to bed, e.g. 'I was laid up for three months'.

To be looking up – to improve.

To be off sick, to be on the sick-list – to be absent from work due to illness.

To be on the mend – to improve.

To be nesh, to be soft – to be prone to illness.

To be under a doctor – to be in a doctor's care.

To find one's legs – to begin to walk after an illness.

To get a chit from the doctor – to get a medical certificate.

To go under – to have an anaesthetic.

To have a bad turn – to become ill suddenly.

To have a bug, a germ – to catch a virus.

To have a check-up – to be medically examined.

To have a set-back – to have a relapse.

To have a temperature – to be feverish, to have a high temperature, e.g. 'I've had a temperature all day'.

To have gas – to have an anaesthetic.

To have painkillers – to have analgesics.

To have sleeping pills – to have sedatives.

To have time off – to have sick leave.

To stitch – to suture.

To suck lozenges – to suck small tablets, usually for coughs and sore throat.

To take a turn for the better – to improve.

To take medicine for the bowels – to take an aperient (the patient uses the word laxative most).

To take stitches out – to remove sutures.

To turn the corner – to improve.

REPRODUCTIVE ORGANS AND SEXUAL PROBLEMS

Gynaecology

The vocabulary to express menstruation and pregnancy is listed separately under Bodily Functions on pages 188–191.

Dilatation and curettage – *D & C*, a scrape, 'I've had two D & Cs' (two scrapes).

Dysmenorrhoea – period pains, to be unwell.

Flooding – excessive bleeding from womb during menopause (or miscarriage).

Hot flushes, to have – to have a high temperature and red face owing to the menopause.

Hysterectomy – to have an internal operation, to have a major operation, to have all taken away (uterus and ovaries).

Menarche – the beginning of periods, e.g. 'When did your periods start'?

Menopause – the end of periods, e.g. 'When did your periods end?', the change, that certain age, the time of life.
I haven't seen anything for six months.
It's your age. It's the time of life.

Repair of the prolapse – 'I was stitched up below', to be hitched up.

Sanitary towels – Pads, STs, Tampax (tampon worn internally), towels, wings.

Vaginal discharge – to have whites, to lose down there. 'Something comes away from me…'

Obstetrics

Confinement – childbirth, delivery. 'Did you have an easy confinement?'

Episiotomy – to make a cut. 'I'm going to cut you now.'

Parturition – labour, to be in labour. 'How often are you having pains?'

Placenta – the afterbirth.

Rupture the membranes, to – to break my waters.

Still-born baby – baby born dead.
Suture – to be stitched up.
Version – turning (of foetus).

Termination of pregnancy

Abortion – spontaneous miscarriage, a miscarriage, a miss*. 'It came away.' 'I lost my baby.'
Medical termination of pregnancy – an abortion. 'I don't want this baby. Can I have an abortion?' 'I did away with it.'* 'I decided, not to go ahead with the pregnancy.'
Efforts to terminate a pregnancy – to bring on a period, to lose it (a baby), to get rid of a baby. 'They took the baby away.'

Sexual expressions

Anal intercourse – buggery, bumming*. 'He wants to come at me from behind.'* to rim*.
Dyspareunia – *love pain.*
A French kiss – kiss with mouth open and insert tongue in partner's mouth.
Illegitimate, to be – to be a bastard, to be born on the wrong side of the blanket, to get into trouble (unmarried pregnancy), to have a natural child.
Oral sex – blow job*, give head*, to go down on someone, rimming, sixty-nine* (mutual oral sex), to suck off.
Orgasm – climax.
  To experience an orgasm: *to come,* to have a thrill.
  'When I come.'
  'When he's finished.'
Sexual intercourse – intimacy, to do it, to fuck*, to get it with, to get layed, to go with someone, *to go to bed with someone,* to have it, *to have sex,* to knock up*, *to make love,* to perform, to shag*, to roger, to screw*, *to sleep with.*
To masturbate – to beat off*, to bring oneself off*, to fiddle*, to jack off*, to jerk off*, to rub up*, to shag*, to shake*, to toss*, to wank*, (wanker: masturbator).

To neck – hug and kiss intimately.

To pet – kiss and caress extensively.

Sexual intercourse is often referred to as *a normal married life* by older people. Note the negative use, such as 'We can't have a normal married life'. Also 'He doesn't trouble me', meaning the husband/partner does not demand sexual intercourse if the woman doesn't want it. 'He doesn't bother about that sort of thing' implies a not very demanding partner. 'He wants it too often' means a demanding one.

Phrases such as, '*When I go with my husband*', *When we have it*', '*When we have sex*', 'When he does it' are most commonly used by ordinary people.

Male expressions

Coitus interruptus – *to be careful*, to withdraw. 'My husband's very careful.'

Ejaculate, to – to come, to get your rocks off*, to shoot.

Erection, to have an – to have a hard on*, to have a stand*, to have a stiff*, to have the horn*.

Impotent, to be – to have a half-stand*. 'I can't keep it up.' 'My husband has trouble.'

Impotent, to become – to lose one's nature.

Semen – come, cum, jizz.

Sexual relations

To have a regular sexual partner – to go steady. 'We're an item.'

Homo and heterosexual – AC – DC*, to be double-jointed*.

Male homosexual – bent, to be a cissy, a dandy, a fag*, a faggot*, a fairy*, a nancy-boy, a pansy, a pouf, a poufter*, a queen, a *queer, gay*, kinky.

Homosexual expressions – to be the active/passive partner, eating ass*, reaming*, tonguing (using the mouth on anus), finger fucking*, fisting* (using finger/fist in anus).

Female homosexual/lesbian – to be gay, kinky, to be butch (a lesbian with male characteristics), a dyke, a lessie.

Family planning

Contraceptives

Condom – briefs (short condoms), Durex (trade name often used as a synonym), envelope, French letter, Johnny*, jolly bag*, rubber*, sheath, skin.

Diaphragm – Dutch cap, cap.

Female condom.

Intrauterine contraceptive devices (IUCDs) – the coil.

Oral contraceptive – the pill.

Sponge.

Fertility clinic

Doctor: *'How often do you try for a baby?* When and how often do you have intercourse?

Tubal insufflation – *I had my tubes blown.*

Seminal fluid – your husband's fluid.

Venereal disease (VD)

Gonorrhoea – clap, gleet, morning drop, strain, tear, a dose, the whites, to catch a cold.

Monilia – Thrush.

Primary syphilis – bumps (West Indian).

Syphilis – bad blood, lues, siff, pox.

Expressions:

To have a double event (syphilis and gonorrhoea).

To piss pins and needles*.

Scalded (infected with gonorrhoea).

Expressions used by patients:

I've been to the GUM clinic.

I've picked up something.

I'm afraid I've got it.

I've caught (or got) something.

I've got a dose (gonorrhoea).

I've got a full house* (syphilis and gonorrhoea).

I've got genital warts.
I've got trouble down below.
I've noticed something odd.
I've got trouble with my meat*.
I've been after the girls (or men).
Lice in pubic hair: to be chatty*, to have crabs*.

Note: 'The whites' may be used by women to mean any white vaginal discharge.

West Indians use 'scratch' for irritate or itch, i.e. 'it scratches me' means 'it irritates and I want to scratch'.

Prostitutes may say, 'I'm a business girl', 'I'm on the game'.

The doctor in a VD clinic will ask: *Have you any discharge? Does it irritate? Do you have pain when you pass water? Have you any swelling? Have you a sore place? Have you a rash?*

Abbreviations used
GUM–Genital Urethral Medicine
FTAT–Fluorescent Treponemal Antibody Test.
STS–Serum Test for Syphilis.
TPI–Treponemal Immobilization Test.
VDRL–Venereal Disease Research Laboratory.
VDRT–Venereal Disease Reference Test.

Idioms

8

PARTS OF THE BODY

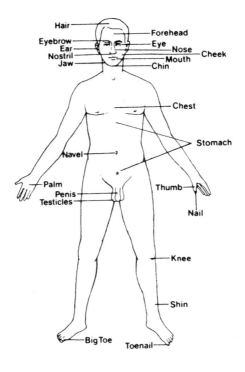

Fig. 1

---

*As used colloquially by patient and often referred to as *tummy*.

IDIOMS

The English language has thousands of idioms. By an idiom we mean a number of words which, when taken together, have a different meaning from that of each separate word.

The reason for including these idioms of parts of the body is that although you may never need to *use* them yourself, you should be able to *recognise* them. You may be told by a patient that by the end of the day he is 'on his knees' and you must realise that he is using the word 'knee' idiomatically. What he means is that he is extremely tired after work and feels like collapsing.

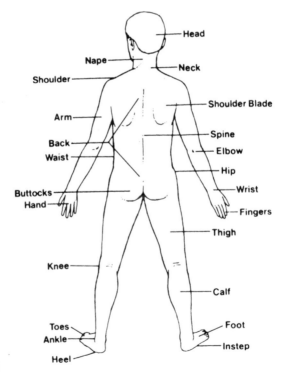

Fig. 2

A woman may tell you of her worries and say she has just managed to 'keep her head above water'. If you are not familiar with the idiom, you may think she has tried to save herself from drowning but, in fact, she means that she is terribly short of money and is having a struggle to keep out of debt.

Words and phrases connected with parts of the body have also been included, such as, chesty, throaty and to speak through one's nose. It is essential that you understand these.

It should be noticed that under 'Nail' appear several idioms which refer to other meanings of the word than the nail of the body. They have been included because they are all commonly used and you should be familiar with them.

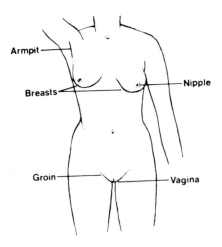

Fig. 3

Arm

A shot in the arm: something that does a person good.
To give one's right arm (usually with *would*): to be willing to make a sacrifice to get something.
To keep someone at arm's length: to avoid being friendly.

To stand by with folded arms: to do nothing when action seems necessary.

To welcome someone with open arms: to greet warmly.

Back

To back a horse: to place money on a horse in a race, to bet.

To back down: to be less demanding than before; to withdraw one's claim.

To back out: to withdraw from.

To back someone or something: to give one's support.

To be on one's back: to be ill in bed.

To break one's back: to overwork.

To do something behind someone's back: to act deceitfully.

To have one's back to the wall: to be struggling against great difficulties.

To put, (get, set) someone's back up: to make someone angry.

To see the back of someone/something: to get rid of someone/something that is annoying, unpleasant.

To turn one's back on: to abandon, to refuse to help.

Blood

A young blood: dashing young man.

Bad blood: ill feeling, (between people, nations).

Blood is thicker than water: one's own relations come before all other people.

His blood is up: he is in a fighting mood.

His blood ran cold in his veins: he was filled with terror.

It is more than flesh and blood can stand: too much for human beings to endure.

One's own flesh and blood: one's own family.

To do something in cold blood: deliberately; when one is not angry.

To get blood out of a stone: to get pity from someone hard; to achieve the impossible.

To get someone's blood up: to provoke someone very much.

To have fresh, new blood: to have new members in a business, family or society.

To make one's blood boil: to make one very angry.

To run in the blood: to have an inherited quality.

Bone

A bone of contention: the subject of constant disagreement.

He will never make old bones: will not live to an old age.

To be all skin and bones: very thin.

To be bone dry: completely dry.

To be bone-idle: completely idle, lazy.

To bone up on: to study intensively.

To feel something in one's bones: to feel quite sure about something intuitively.

To have a bone to pick with someone: to wish to complain about something.

To make no bones about doing something: to have no hesitation in doing something (usually unpleasant).

To work one's fingers to the bone: to work very hard without appreciation.

Brain

A brain-child: original idea of a person or group.

A brain-drain: movement of trained and qualified workers to other countries (usually for better conditions).

A brain-storm: cerebral disturbance; a mental aberration.

A brain-storming session: a method of solving problems in which many people suggest ideas which are then discussed.

A brain-teaser: problem, puzzle.

A brain-wave: a sudden inspiration or clever idea.

A scatter-brained person: a careless, forgetful person.

Brain-fag: mental exhaustion.

Brain fever: encephalitis.

Brain-washing: forcing someone to change his beliefs by use of extreme mental pressure.

Brainless: foolish, stupid.

Brainy: clever.

To blow one's brain out: to shoot oneself in the head.

To have something on the brain: to be obsessive about something.

To pick someone's brains: to find out someone's good ideas and use them.

To rack one's brains: to think very hard; to solve a problem or remember something.

Breast

To make a clean breast of something: to confess everything.

Brow (forehead), Brows (arch of hair above eyes)

A high-brow: someone interested in intellectual matters and culture.

A low-brow: someone showing little interest in intellectual matters and culture.

To browbeat someone into doing something: to intimidate someone with severe looks and words, bully.

To knit one's brows: to frown.

Cheek

Cheek: disrespectful speech, impudence.

Cheeks: buttocks.

To be cheeky: to be disrespectful, impudent.

To cheek someone: to speak impudently to someone.

To have the cheek to do something: to be bold, rude enough to do something.

To turn the other cheek: to refuse to retaliate.

Chest

To be chesty: to have trouble with one's lungs.

To cock one's chest: to boast about oneself.

To get something off one's chest: to free one's mind by speaking about something that was troubling one.

Get that across your chest! Eat that! (usually a large, nourishing meal).

To puff one's chest out: to be proud of oneself.

Chin

A chin: a talk.

Chin up: be brave.

To be up to the chin in work, etc.: to have too much work to do.

To chin: to talk, gossip.

To have a chin-wag: to talk with friends about unimportant matters; to chatter.

To keep one's chin up: to be brave, to be cheerful in the face of difficulties.

To take something on the chin: to suffer severe difficulties with courage.

Ears

To be all ears: to listen very carefully.

To be up to one's ears in: deeply involved or occupied in.

To box someone's ears: to smack someone on the ears.

To come to one's ears: to hear a rumour.

To earmark: to put someone/something aside for a special purpose.

To fall on deaf ears: to pass unnoticed.

To give one's ears for something: to be prepared to do anything to get what one desires.

In at one ear and out at the other: ignored or quickly forgotten advice.

To have a person's ear: to have the favourable attention of someone.

To have a word in someone's ear: to speak in private.

To keep one's ear to the ground: to listen carefully.

To play it by ear: to do what seems best at the time.

To prick up one's ears: to have one's attention suddenly aroused.

To send someone away with a flea in his ear: to criticise someone severely so that he goes away unhappily.

To set people by the ears: to cause them to quarrel.

To turn a deaf ear: to ignore, pretend not to hear.

Elbow

Elbow-grease: vigorous polishing; hard work.

Elbow-room: plenty of room to move freely.

Out-at-elbows: of a coat, worn out; of a person, poor.

To elbow one's way through a crowd: to push with one's elbows.

To raise the elbow: to drink too much.

Eye

A blue-eyed boy: a pet, favourite.

A sight for sore eyes: someone or something very welcome, pleasant.

A sore eye: an inflamed eye.

An eye for an eye: to punish those who hurt us.

An eye-opener: an event or piece of news which causes surprise.

An eyesore: a very unpleasant thing to look at.

Eyeball to eyeball: face to face with someone.

Eye contact: looking directly into another person's eyes.

Eye-opener: an enlightening experience.

Eye-wash: lotion for bathing eyes; words or actions intended to mislead.

Green-eyed: jealous.

In the eyes of: in the opinion of.

In the mind's eye: imagining in the mind.

In the public eye: to be watched by the public constantly.

The apple of one's eye: someone or something very precious.

To be up to the eyes in work: to have far too much work to do.

To catch someone's eye: to attract someone's attention.

To cry one's eyes out: to weep very much.

To do something with one's eyes open: to act knowing the results of the action.

To eye someone: to look at carefully, admiringly, jealously, etc.

To get (or give) a black eye: to receive (or give) a blow on the eye so that the skin around it goes black.

To give someone the glad eye: to encourage someone to be amorous.

To have an eye for: to have a liking or ability to do something; to have good judgement on something.

To have an eye on/to the main chance: to think and work with one's own advantage always in view.

To have half an eye on: not to give something one's full attention.

To have one's eyes opened: to be forced to see reality.

To keep an eye on someone/something: to watch carefully.

To keep one's eye open for: to watch carefully.

To keep one's eyes skinned: to be very watchful.

To make eyes at someone: to look at someone (usually of the opposite sex) with open admiration and invitation.

To pull the wool over someone's eyes: to try to hide the truth from someone.

To run one's eye over: to look quickly at, to glance at.

To see eye to eye with someone: to agree; to have the same ideas.

To turn a blind eye: to ignore deliberately, pretend not to see.

Face

Face-ache: neuralgia.

Let's face it: let's be honest with each other.

To be a slap in the face: a sudden disappointment, rejection.

To face the music: to face criticism/punishment as a result of one's own actions.

To face up to something: to meet courageously (usually difficulties).

To fly in the face of convention, rules, etc.: to defy, disobey openly.

To have a face as long as a fiddle: to look depressed.

To keep a straight face: not laugh. (Often used negatively – e.g. 'I couldn't keep a straight face'.)

To look someone in the face: to look directly at someone.

To lose face: to be humiliated, to be put to shame.

To make/pull a face: to grimace.

To pull a long face: to look depressed, disappointed, displeased.

To put a brave/good face on it: to behave as if circumstances are better than they really are.

To put one's face on: to apply cosmetics to one's face.

To save one's face: to try to avoid shaming oneself openly.

To set one's face against: to oppose.

To show one's face: to appear, be seen.

To stare one in the face: something that is obvious, clear to see.

Feet – see Foot

Fingers

Not to raise (lift, stir) a finger to help someone: to refuse to be of any help.

One's fingers itch to do something: one wishes very much to do something.

To be all fingers and thumbs: to be clumsy with one's hands often due to nervousness.

To be light-fingered: to steal easily.

To burn one's fingers: to get into trouble by interfering in other people's affairs.

To finger: to touch.

To get/pull one's finger out: to stop being lazy, work harder (slang).

To have a finger in every pie: to be involved in many activities.

To have butter-fingers: to let things slip out of the hands.

To have something at one's finger-tips: to know perfectly.

To keep one's fingers crossed (for someone): hope for luck with a problem or difficulty.

To lay/put one's finger on something: to realise the most important aspect of a matter.

To let something slip through one's fingers: to lose hold of, allow to escape (usually of opportunities).

To twist a person round one's finger: to have someone in one's power so that they do all one wishes.

Flesh

Flesh wound: one not reaching bone or a vital organ.

One's own flesh and blood: one's own family.

Proud flesh: new flesh coming from a wound.

Sins of the flesh: sexual sins.

To be neither fish nor flesh: to be of indefinite character.

To have one's pound of flesh: to insist cruelly on repayment.

To lose flesh: to get thinner.

To make one's flesh creep: to be terrified so that one's skin seems to move.

To put on flesh: to get fatter.

To see someone in the flesh: actually to see someone.

Foot, Feet

My foot!: Nonsense! Rubbish!

Not to let the grass grow under one's feet: to act quickly when one has made a decision.

To be on one's feet: to be in reasonable health; to be standing.

To be run off one's feet: to be so busy one cannot sit down.

To dog one's footsteps: to follow one constantly and so cause irritation.

To drag one's feet: to be slow to take action.

To fall on one's feet: to be lucky.

To fall over one's feet to be kind, helpful, etc.: to make a great effort.

To find one's feet: to be comfortably settled in a new job, situation, etc.

To foot the bill: to pay.

To get cold feet: to be afraid, discouraged.

To go on foot: to walk.

To have one foot in the grave: to be very ill, close to death.

To have one's feet on the ground: to be practical, sensible.

To have the world at one's feet: to be very successful.

To put one's best foot forward: to walk quickly, to work quickly.

To put one's feet up: to relax, rest.

To put one's foot down: to be firm, protest.

To put one's foot in it: to do or say something that causes anger, trouble.

To set someone on his feet: to help, usually with money, to start a business, etc.

To stand on one's own feet: to be independent.

To step off on the wrong foot: to start something in the wrong way.

Hair

A hair's breadth: a very small distance.

Hair-raising (stories): terrifying.

Not turn a hair: to show no sign of fear or emotional upset.

To a hair: exactly (usually of weight).

To get in a person's hair: to annoy, irritate someone.

To have one's hair standing on end: to be terrified.

To have someone by the short hairs: to have control over them.

To keep one's hair on: not to grow angry.

To let down one's hair: to act freely, to be uninhibited.

To split hairs: to argue about very small, unimportant differences.

Hand

A right-hand man: someone who can be relied on for help and advice.

At first hand: directly.

Hands off!: Do not touch.

Hands on experience: involving active participation.

Never to do a hand's turn: never make the slightest effort.

To be a handful: to be difficult to control.

To be an old hand at something: to be experienced.

To be hand-in-glove with someone: to be extremely friendly (usually planning something together).

To be high-handed: to be arrogant.

To be off-hand: to be abrupt in manner, casual.

To be off one's hands: to be no longer responsible for someone or something.

To be open-handed: to be generous with money.

To be out of hand (of children, a situation, etc.): to be out of control.

To be under-hand: to be deceitful, dishonest, not open.

To eat out of someone's hand: to do whatever one wishes.

To force someone's hand: to make someone do something.

To get one's hand in: to get to know how to do something.

To give/lend someone a hand: to help someone physically.

To give someone a free hand: to allow someone to do as he wishes.

To hand: to give, to offer.

To have a hand in something: to share in the activity.

To have one's hands full: to be extremely busy.

To have one's hands tied: to be unable to act in the way one wishes.

To have the upper hand over someone: to dominate.

To have time on one's hands: to have plenty of free time.

To keep one's hand in: to be in practice.

To lay hands on: to seize, touch (often used negatively).

To live from hand to mouth: to live from day to day; without regular money.

To play into someone's hands: to do something which helps one's opponent.

To rule with a heavy hand: to rule severely.

To say off-hand: to give an answer immediately from memory.

To take one's courage in both hands: to force oneself to do something difficult, unpleasant.

To take someone in hand: to try to improve someone's behaviour.

To try one's hand at something: to make an attempt to do something new.

To wait on someone hand and foot: to attend to someone's needs with great care.

To wash one's hands of someone/something: to have nothing more to do with.

Head

A headache: a pain in the head; a difficult problem; a troublesome person.

From head to foot/toe: completely; all over the person.

It is on his head: he is responsible for it.

Not to know whether one is standing on one's head or one's heels: to be in a state of extreme confusion.

To be big-headed: to be conceited.

To be block-headed: to be dull, stupid.

To be fat-headed: to be stupid.

To be hard-headed: to be practical, unsentimental.

To be head and shoulders above others: to be much taller; to be far superior.

To be head over heels in love: completely, very much.

To be hot-headed: to be hasty, impulsive.

To be above/over one's head: too difficult to understand.

To be pig-headed: to be obstinate.

To be soft-headed: to be simple-minded.

To be touched in the head: to be slightly mad.

To bite a person's head off: to speak sharply, angrily to someone.

To bury one's head in the sand: to avoid facing facts by pretending not to see them.

To come to a head: to reach a crisis.

To eat one's head off: to eat an excessive amount.

To get something into one's head: be convinced that something is true.

To get one's head down: to go to bed.

To go off one's head: to become crazy, mad.

To go to one's head: to make one excited, to intoxicate one.

To have a good head for business: to have a natural aptitude for it.

To have a good head-piece: to have plenty of brains.

To have a head: to have a headache, often from drinking too much.

To have a head like a sieve: to be very forgetful.

To have an old head on young shoulders: to be wise beyond one's years.

To have one's head screwed on the right way: to be intelligent, full of common sense, especially in practical matters.

To have something hanging over one's head: to have some danger, something unpleasant going to happen soon.

To head off: to divert a person from someone or something.

To heap coals of fire on a person's head: to treat a person well who has treated oneself badly.

To hit the nail on the head: to guess right, to reach the correct conclusion.

To keep one's head: to stay calm in a difficult situation.

To keep one's head above water: to keep out of debt.

To knock on the head: to destroy, disrupt an idea, plan, etc.

To let someone have his head: to let him do as he wishes.

To lose one's head: to lose one's self-control in a difficult situation.

To make head, headway: to make progress.

To make head or tail of something: to understand it. (Usually used negatively: 'I couldn't make head or tail of the letter he sent me'.)

To put something out of one's head: to forget it deliberately, to stop thinking about it.

To put things into someone's head: to suggest things to him.

To run/knock one's head against a stone wall: to do something that will fail, because of opposition.

To take it into one's head: to make a sudden decision.

To talk someone's head off: to talk so much that the other person is weary.

Two heads are better than one: two people know more together than one person.

Heart

After one's own heart: a person sharing one's own interests, opinions.

At heart: basically, deep down.

Have a heart! Be reasonable; don't be unkind!

Heartache: deep sorrow, grief.

Heartburn: pain in chest as a result of indigestion, pyrosis.

Heart-felt sympathy: deepest sympathy.

Heart-searching: doubts, uncertainties.

In one's heart of hearts: deep down in oneself.

Not to have the heart to do something: not to have the courage to do something.

The heart of the matter: the essence, the vital part.

To be down-hearted: to be depressed.

To be good at heart: to be good basically.

To be half-hearted about something: not to be very enthusiastic.

To be hard-hearted: to be hard, unkind.

To be heartless: to be unkind, unsympathetic.

To be hearty: to be cheerful.

To be in good heart: to be cheerful, confident.

To be lion-hearted: to be very brave.

To be soft-hearted: to be kind, sympathetic.

To be stout-hearted: to be very brave.

To break one's heart: to be overwhelmed with sorrow.

To cause heartache: to cause suffering.

To cry one's heart out: to cry excessively.

To eat one's heart out: to fret, worry excessively.

To have a big heart: to be warm, generous.

To have a heart-to-heart talk with someone: to speak openly, hiding nothing.

To have a hearty appetite: to have a very good appetite.

To have no heart: to be hard, insensitive.

To have no heart for something: to have no enthusiasm for something.

To have one's heart in one's boots: to be depressed, to feel hopeless.

To have one's heart in one's mouth: to be very afraid.

To know, learn, say by heart: to know word for word by memory.

To lose heart: to have no hope, to become discouraged, (often used negatively): 'Don't lose heart: keep on hoping'.

To lose one's heart: to fall in love.

To put one's heart into something: to do something with enthusiasm.

To set one's heart on something: to want something very much.

To take heart: to become more hopeful.

To take someone to one's heart: to feel deep affection for someone.

To take something to heart: to be upset; to worry too much about things.

To tear one's heart-strings: to hurt one very deeply.

Whole-hearted: complete, without doubts.

Heel(s)

A heel: a completely unreliable person.

An/one's Achilles heel: weak or vulnerable point, especially of character.

Not to know whether one is standing on one's head or one's heels: to be in a state of extreme confusion.

To be down at heel: poorly dressed and in a state of poverty.

To be head over heels in love: completely, very much.

To bring someone to heel: to put under control.

To carry with the heels first: as a dead body.

To come on the heels of: to follow immediately.

To kick one's heels: to stand waiting idly, impatiently.

To leave to cool his heels: to make someone wait deliberately.

To show a clean pair of heels: to run away.

To take to one's heels: to run away.

Knee

To be knee-deep in something: deeply involved in.

To be on one's knees: to kneel, especially when praying; to be completely exhausted.

To bring someone to his knees: to make him submit, stop fighting.

To go down on one's knees to someone: to beg for something.

To have a knees-up: a very lively party.

Knuckles

To knuckle down to a job: to work as hard as one can.

To knuckle under: to accept defeat.

To rap someone's knuckles: to reprimand.

Lap (waist to knees of one sitting)

In the lap of the gods: uncertain future.

In the lap of luxury: in great comfort and luxury.

Leg

A blackleg: a person who continues working when others are on strike.

Not to have a leg to stand on: have no good reason to support one's argument.

The boot is on the other leg: the truth is the opposite of what one believes.

To be on one's last legs: to be close to death; utterly weary.

To find one's legs: to be able to stand and walk (usually after an illness).

To get one's sea-legs: to become used to the movement of a ship.

To give someone a leg up: to help someone.

To pull someone's leg: to tease someone.

To show a leg: to get out of bed.

To stretch one's legs: to go for a walk.

To walk someone off his legs: to tire him out with walking.

Lip

Lip: saucy talk, impudence.

None of your lip!: Don't speak to me like that.

Lip-language, reading, speaking: use of the movement of the lips to and by the deaf and dumb.

A word escapes one's lips: something is said without thought.

To bite one's lip: to stop oneself from saying something; to hide emotion.

To curl one's lip: to show scorn.

To hang on someone's lip: to listen with great care.

To have sealed lips: to be silent about something.

To keep a stiff upper lip: to bear troubles without showing emotion.

To lick one's lips: to show appreciation of food (or sometimes other things).

To pay lip service to principles, etc.: to say one believes in something but not to act accordingly.

Mind

Mind: memory, remembrance.

Mind-blowing: (of drugs, etc.) causing ecstasy, excitement; (of news) confusing, shattering.

Mind-boggling: astonishing, extraordinary; overwhelming.

Never mind: It doesn't matter; don't worry.

To be not in one's right mind: to be mad.

To be out of one's mind: to be mad.

To bear something in mind: to remember.

To bend someone's mind: to influence the mind so that it is permanently affected.

To give someone a piece of one's mind: to speak openly and critically.

To go out of one's mind: to go mad: 'He went out of his mind in the end'; to be forgotten: 'I'm so sorry. It went out of my mind'.

To have presence of mind: to act and think quickly in emergencies.

To have something on one's mind: to be worried about something.

To know one's own mind: to be definite about what one wants.

To make up one's mind: to decide.

To mind: (a) to be careful (used very often in orders): 'Mind the step' – be careful of the step; 'Mind the car' – get out of the way of the car. (b) to care (often used negatively): 'I don't mind what she does or says'. (c) to object (used mainly interrogatively and negatively): 'I don't mind going to hospital to have my baby'. Note the polite request: 'Would you mind' + -ing form of the verb: 'Would you mind lying on the couch?'. (d) to take care of: 'She had no-one to mind the baby when she went to work'. Noun: a baby-minder.

To mind one's own business: not to interfere in the affairs of other people.

To mind one's p's and q's: to be careful what one says and does.

To mind out for: avoid.

To take a load/weight off someone's mind: cause great relief.

Mouth

Mouth: impudent talk, rudeness.

To be down in the mouth: to be depressed.

To look as if butter would not melt in one's mouth: to look innocent, incapable of badness.

To make one's mouth water: to cause saliva to flow at the sight of food.

To put words into someone's mouth: to tell someone what to say.

To take the words out of someone's mouth: to say what someone was about to say.

Nail(s)

Nail-biting: causing anxiety or tension.

To be as hard as nails: to be very tough; merciless.

To be as right as nails: to be perfectly fit.

To fight tooth and nail: to fight fiercely, vigorously.

To hit the nail on the head: to say the right thing; guess right.

To nail someone down: to make someone give a definite statement; details.

To pay on the nail: to pay at once.

To put a nail in one's coffin: to do something that will shorten one's life.

Neck

Neck: boldness, disrespect, impertinence.

Neck or nothing: desperately risking everything for success.

Stiff-necked: obstinate, proud, stubborn.

To be a pain in the neck: to be a nuisance and pest to someone.

To be up to the neck in debt, work: to be completely immersed in.

To break one's neck to do something: work extremely hard to do something.

To get it in the neck: to be severely punished.

To have the neck to do something: to be rude enough to do something.

To neck: to hug and kiss someone intimately.

To run neck and neck: to be level with someone in a competition.

To save one's neck: to save oneself from punishment.

To stick one's neck out: to act or speak in a way which exposes one to harm or criticism.

To talk out of the back of one's neck: to talk nonsense.

To throw someone out neck and crop: to throw someone out head first, bodily.

Nerve(s)

Nerve-racking: frightening, stressful.

Not to know what nerves are: to have a calm temperament.

To be a bundle of nerves: in a very nervous state.

To get on one's nerves: to annoy or irritate very much.

To have a fit of nerves: to be in a nervous state.

To have iron/steel nerves: not to be easily upset or frightened.

To have the nerve to do something: to be brave, to be impudent enough.

To lose one's nerve: to become frightened and unsure of oneself.

To nerve oneself to do something: to use all one's strength, mental and physical.

To strain every nerve: to make a great effort.

What a nerve!: What impudence!

Nose

To cut off one's nose to spite one's face: to do something in anger to hurt someone else which also hurts oneself.

To follow one's nose: to go straight on; to act on instinct.

To get up a person's nose: to annoy someone.

To have a good nose: to have a good sense of smell.

To keep one's nose to the grindstone: to work hard over a long period.

To lead someone by the nose: to make someone do anything one wishes.

To look down one's nose at someone: to regard someone as inferior.

To nose about: to look enquiringly everywhere.

To pay through the nose: to pay an excessive price.

To poke one's nose into something: to try to find out about people and things which do not concern one.

To put someone's nose out of joint: to do something to irritate or upset someone.

To see no further than one's nose: not to be able to imagine the future or any situation other than the current one.

To speak through one's nose: to speak with a nasal sound (often as a result of adenoids).

To turn up one's nose: to show dislike or disapproval.

Palm

To grease someone's palm: to bribe him, offer money for information, etc.

To palm something off on someone: to sell something that is worthless or damaged.

Shoulder

A shoulder to cry on: someone who listens to one's problems with sympathy.

Shoulder to shoulder: with united effort.

Straight from the shoulder: a strong blow or strong criticism of someone.

To cold-shoulder someone: to ignore someone deliberately; treat coldly.

To have a chip on one's shoulder: to go around with a sense of grievance.

To have an old head on young shoulders: a young person who is wise beyond his age.

To have broad shoulders: to be strong; to be able to bear responsibility.

To put one's shoulder to the wheel: to make a great effort to do something.

To rub shoulders with: to mix with people.

To shoulder (a burden or the blame): to carry.

Skin

Skin-deep: (of beauty, emotion, wound), no deeper than the skin, not lasting, on the surface.

A skinflint: a mean, miserly person.

A skinhead: a member of a group of young people who have closely-cut hair, strange clothes and are often violent.

To be skin and bone: very thin.

To be thick-skinned: not to care what others say about one, insensitive.

To be thin-skinned: to be too sensitive to what others say.

To escape by the skin of one's teeth: to have a narrow escape.

To get under one's skin: to annoy intensely; to hold one's interest very much.

To jump out of one's skin: to be startled, frightened suddenly.

To keep one's eyes skinned: to be watchful.

To save one's skin: to avoid or escape from danger.

To skin: for a wound to be covered with new skin; to remove skin from something.

Skull

Thick-skulled: dull, stupid person.

To get something into one's skull: to understand and remember it.

Stomach

To have a strong stomach: ability not to feel nausea; can eat anything.

To have butterflies in the stomach: to have fluttery feelings in the stomach due to nervousness.

To stomach something: accept (usually in negative form). 'He cannot stomach her ways'; cannot bear them.

To turn one's stomach: cause someone to be disgusted.

Teeth — see Tooth

Throat

Cut-throat competition: fierce, intense struggle in business.

Throaty: guttural, spoken in the throat.

To cut one's own throat: to act in a way that harms oneself; to kill oneself.

To have a frog in one's throat: hoarseness or loss of voice.

To have a lump in one's throat: to feel choked with emotion so that one can hardly speak.

To have a throat: to have a sore throat.

To have words stick in one's throat: to be too embarrassed by something to be able to speak of it.

To jump down someone's throat: to speak angrily to someone.

To thrust something down someone's throat: to try to make someone accept one's own beliefs, views, etc.

Thumb

Thumbs up!: mark of victory, satisfaction.

To be under someone's thumb: to be dominated by someone.

To thumb a lift: to sign with the thumb to ask a motorist for a free lift.

To twiddle one's thumbs: to have to sit still and do nothing.

Toe(s)

From top to toe: from head to foot, completely.

To be on one's toes: to be ready for action, alert.

To step/tread on someone's toes: to annoy someone unwittingly (often by doing what they want to do).

To tiptoe: to walk on the tips of one's toes; to walk quietly.

To toe the line: to obey the rules, of a party, society, etc.

To turn up one's toes: to die.

Tongue

A slip of the tongue: a mistake made when speaking.

Tongue: language, e.g. one's mother tongue: one's native language.

To be tongue-tied: to be too shy, too nervous to speak.

To have a dangerous tongue: to speak maliciously.

To have a long tongue: to be talkative.

To have a ready tongue: to speak easily, fluently.

To have something on the tip of one's tongue: to be about to say something and then forget it.

To hold one's tongue: to be silent.

To lose one's tongue: to be too shy to speak.

To put out one's tongue: grimace to mark displeasure; for doctor's inspection.

To speak with one's tongue in one's cheek: to say something which is not true in order to joke with someone.

To wag one's tongue: to talk indiscreetly, to gossip.

Tooth, Teeth

In the teeth of evidence, opposition, wind, etc.: against it.

Teething troubles: difficulties in the first stages of something.

To be armed to the teeth: to be fully armed with many weapons.

To be fed up to the back teeth with something: to be bored by, tired of.

To be long in the tooth: to be old.

To cast something in someone's teeth: to blame him for it.

To cut a tooth: a new tooth begins to show above the gum (of babies and children).

To cut one's eye-teeth: to gain worldly wisdom, maturity.

To cut one's wisdom teeth: (as to cut one's eye-teeth).

To escape by the skin of one's teeth: to have a narrow escape.

To fight tooth and nail: to fight with all one's strength.

To get one's teeth into something: to make an enthusiastic start on a job, etc.

To have a sweet tooth: to enjoy eating sweet things.

To set one's teeth on edge: to cause an unpleasant feeling in the teeth; to cause disgust.

To show one's teeth: to become aggressive.

To take the bit between one's teeth: to reject the advice and control of others.

Phrasal verbs

Phrasal verb is a name given to those combinations of verb plus preposition or adverbial particle from which we have now hundreds of phrases to describe everyday events and activities.

The most commonly used phrasal verbs are formed from the shortest and simplest verbs in the English language such as come, do, get, go, make, put, take, followed by words such as down, from, in, out, up and to. A phrasal verb consists of two (sometimes three) parts and it is essential to consider the parts together, for the combination often makes a different meaning. Some phrasal verbs have several meanings.

Those who study the English language have great difficulty in understanding and using phrasal verbs correctly. For this reason a whole chapter is given to them. It is quite impossible to follow everyday speech without a knowledge of phrasal verbs, because we use them in preference to more formal words. To take some examples: we talk about 'getting up' in the morning and 'putting our clothes on' rather than 'rising' and 'dressing'.

Doctors must use language understood easily by their patients, so they ask, for example, 'When did the pain first come on?' meaning onset of pain, or say 'I want you to cut down on fatty foods', meaning reduce intake. The examples given here are mostly taken from the hospital situation and so are invaluable to you.

Many of you reading this book will be working alone, so to help you learn these special verbs there is a test paper with answers.

BREAK

— **Break down:**

    i. *collapse mentally or physically, often due to stress.* Dr Foster worked night and day and eventually his health broke down.

ii. *cry with grief, shock, etc.* If I talk about losing my baby, I break down.

iii. *fail to work because of electrical, mechanical, etc. fault.* The cardiac imaging system has broken down.

iv. *fail, discontinue.* Negotiations over the ambulance workers' pay dispute have broken down.

— **Break in:** *enter somewhere by force.* I could never sleep alone in the house after burglars broke in.

— **Break out:** *sudden start of disease, fire, violence, war.* An epidemic of cholera broke out in the refugee camp.

— **Break out in something:** *suddenly become covered in.* (a) Whenever I eat strawberries I break out in a rash. (b) I keep waking up and breaking out in a cold sweat.

— **Break through:** *make a major discovery or advance.* The pharmaceutical company hopes to break through with a new treatment for Alzheimer's Disease.

— **Break up:** *deteriorate (of health).* He's breaking up under the strain of nursing his wife.

— **Break something up:** *come to end (of relationships).* I've been ill ever since my marriage broke up.

— **Break with:** *end relations with someone.* My son has broken with us since he mixed with this group.

BRING

— **Bring something about:** *cause something to happen.* Drug abuse brought about his death.

— **Bring something back:** *call to mind.* Talking to you brings back memories of my childhood.

— **Bring someone back to something:** *restore.* A complete change will bring you back to health.

— **Bring someone down:** *defeat, degrade.* Heavy drinking brought him down.

— **Bring something down:** *lower, reduce.* Reducing your weight will help to bring down the cholesterol levels in your blood.

— **Bring something on:** *cause.* It would help me to know what brings on your chest pain.

— **Bring someone round:** *restore to consciousness.* The patient was brought round by mouth-to-mouth ventilation.

— **Bring someone through:** *save someone's life.* Her husband was critically ill but the doctors and nurses struggled all night to bring him through and he survived.

— **Bring someone to:** *restore to consciousness.*

— **Bring someone up:** *rear, teach a child social habits* (often used in passive). His mother died when he was two so he was brought up by his grandmother. (Note: to be well brought up. To be badly brought up.)

— **Bring something up:**
　i. *vomit.* She's not well. She brought up her lunch today.
　ii. *eructation.* Do you bring any wind up?

COME

— **Come about:** *happen.* How did the accident come about? He crashed his car in the fog.

— **Come across:** *make an impression of a particular kind.* She comes across as a very nervous woman.

— **Come across someone/something:** *find, meet or see unexpectedly.* I've never come across such a bad case of shingles before.

— **Come along:** *make progress.* You're coming along nicely. We should have those stitches out soon.

— **Come back:** *return.* (a) Make an appointment to come back in a month. (b) my ulcer has come back since I started my new job.

— **Come back to someone:** *return to memory.* Yes, what happened is all coming back to me now. I remember falling down the steps.

— **Come by something:** *get, obtain.* How did you come by that scar on your cheek? I was in a fight and someone threw a bottle at me.

— **Come down (of prices, temperature, etc.):** *be lowered, fall.* Your blood pressure has come down since we started you on the tablets.

— **Come down on someone:** *criticise someone, punish.* The police come down heavily on people found with hard drugs.

— **Come down with something:** *become ill with something.* She came down with flu and was unable to keep her appointment.

— **Come forward:** *present oneself, with help, information, etc.* 'Will anyone who saw the accident please come forward?'

— **Come from:** *have as one's birthplace* (not used in the continuous tenses). Where do you come from? India.

— **Come in:**
   i. *be admitted to hospital.* I'd like your mother to come in so we can do one or two tests.
   ii. *be introduced, begin to be used.* More people were treated quicker and better when day surgery and keyhole surgery came in.

— **Come off something:** *fall from a bicycle, horse, etc.* My son came off his motor bike and broke his left leg.

— **Come on:**
   i. *encourage someone to hurry, make an effort, try harder* (used in imperative only). Come on Mr Hopkins. Let's see you walk across the room now.
   ii. *grow, make progress.* Good. Your baby's coming on very well.
   iii. *start (of symptoms etc.)* Tell me exactly when these panic attacks first came on.

— **Come out:**
   i. *be published.* When's your new book coming out?
   ii. *become known.* It's just come out that they are closing down the factory and I shall lose my job.
   iii. *publicly acknowledge one's homosexuality.* John and Simon have come out.

iv. *stop work, strike*. Do you think doctors and nurses should come out for better working conditions?

— **Come out in something:** *be partially covered in rash, spots, etc*. Her hands came out in a rash after she used a new detergent.

— **Come over:** *begin to feel dizzy, faint, etc*. It's happened twice now travelling home from work. I came over faint.

— **Come round:** *regain consciousness*. Your son hasn't come round yet from the anaesthetic.

— **Come through something:** *recover from a serious illness, accident, survive*. You're lucky to have come through such a terrible accident.

— **Come to:** *regain consciousness*. When I came to, I was on the bathroom floor.

— **Come under something:** *be classified as*. Heroin and cocaine come under Class A of the Misuse of Drugs Act.

— **Come up:**
  i. *arise (of a subject)*. The question of the rights of patients is always coming up these days.
  ii. *happen, occur*. I'm afraid I shall be late for my clinic. Something urgent has come up.

CUT

— **Cut back (on) something:** *reduce expenditure*. Because of financial restrictions, all departments have had to cut back drastically.

— **Cut something down; cut down (on something):** *reduce amount or quantity*. (a) I've already cut my cigarettes down to 10 a day. (b) You must cut down on the fats you eat.

— **Cut someone off:** *break the connection on the telephone* (often used in passive). How annoying. I've just been cut off in the middle of a conversation.

— **Cut something off:**
  i. *amputate, remove*. Following the explosion, the man had to have his left leg cut off.

    ii. *stop the supply of something* (often used in passive). The
    electricity has been cut off.

— **Cut off:** *isolated.* She feels very cut off since she got
cancer.

— **Cut out something:**

    i. *excise.* I had a lump on my neck cut out.

    ii. *stop eating, using.* I've cut out alcohol completely.

— **Cut someone up:** *upset emotionally* (usually in the passive).
He was terribly cut up by his wife's death.

DO

— **Do away with oneself:** *to commit suicide, kill oneself.* I feel so
depressed, Doctor, I could do away with myself.

— **Do someone in:**

    i. *exhaust* (usually in passive). At the end of the week I'm
    absolutely done in.

    ii. *kill* (usually in passive). The old man was done in. (slang)

— **Do something in:** *injure a part of the body.* He did his back in
moving furniture.

— **Do something to something:** *cause something to happen*
(usually with questions with *what.*) What have you done to
your leg? It's bleeding.

— **Do something up:**

    i. *fasten with buttons or zip, etc.* Well, Mr Cox, let's see if you
    can do up your clothes.

    ii. *modernise, redecorate, restore.* These wards are depressing.
    They need doing up.

— **Do with something:**

    i. *be concerned with, connected with* (use with *have to*). His
    job has something to do with medical ethics.

    ii. *need, wish for* (used with *can* and *could*). You could do
    with some new glasses. Go and have your eyes tested.

— **Do without someone/something:** *manage without.* We've
had to do without a speech therapist since the last one left.

FIND

— **Find something out:** *discover the truth, learn some information.* When did you find out your son was on drugs?

FIT

— **Fit someone/something in:** *manage to find time to see someone or do something.* Doctor is booked up all morning but as it's urgent I'll try and fit you in.
— **Fit in with someone/something:** *suit, harmonise with someone/something.* Do you think she will fit in with the rest of the team?
— **Fit someone/something out/up with:** *equip.* These operating rooms are fitted out/up with the latest equipment.

GET

— **Get about:**
   i. *move from place to place.* I can't get about much now that I've got arthritis.
   ii. *spread (of news, rumour).* It got about that doctors might charge for home visits.
— **Get something across:** *communicate something to someone.* It's quite difficult to get across to my mother that she can't go on living alone.
— **Get along:** *make progress.* Fine. You're getting along very well.
— **Get along with someone:** *have a good relationship with somebody.* Do you get along with your family?
— **Get around:** — as for *Get about.*
— **Get at someone:** *criticise someone repeatedly* (usually in continuous tenses). The other children are always getting at him and he's afraid of going to school now.
— **Get at someone/something:**
   i. *reach.* Make sure you put these tablets somewhere where the children can't get at them.

ii. *mean, try to say*. I'm not sure what you're getting at.

— **Get away:** *have a holiday*. You should try to get away for a few days after the operation.

— **Get back:** *arrive, return home*. He says he can get back on his own.

— **Get back to someone:** *contact someone again later*. I don't have the information you need just now but I'll get back to you.

— **Get something back:** *recover something that was lost*. He's now got back the use of his arm which was paralysed by the stroke.

— **Get by:** *manage, cope with life*. Single parent families often have a struggle to get by.

— **Get someone down:** *depress*. All this quarrelling in the family gets me down.

— **Get something down:** *swallow* (with difficulty). The tablets you gave me last time were so big I could hardly get them down.

— **Get into:** *start bad habits*. How did she get into drugs?

— **Get (someone) off:** *fall asleep, help someone to fall asleep*. It takes me ages to get the baby off at night.

— **Get off something:** *leave work with permission*. He got a week off when his wife had a baby.

— **Get on:**
    i. *perform* (often used in questions with *how*). (a) How did you get on in the exam? (b) I got on fine in medicine but I failed in English.
    ii. *progress*. Take these tablets for a month and we'll see how you get on.

— **Get on with someone:** *have a good relationship with*. I get on fine with my children but I don't get on with my wife.

— **Get out:** *leave the house*. You must try to get out more. No wonder you are depressed, sitting here alone all day.

— **Get out of something:**
    i. *escape the necessity or duty to do something*. He managed to get out of working nights for a month.

ii. *give up a habit.* I wish I could get out of the habit of smoking after every meal.

— **Get over something:**

i. *overcome.* No need to worry. I'm sure we can get over that problem.

ii. *recover from disappointment, illness, shock.* He's getting over the shock of losing his wife extremely well.

— **Get something over:** *complete something difficult or unpleasant.* Thank goodness I've got the hysterectomy over.

— **Get something over to someone:** *make someone understand.* You must get over to your husband the importance of remaining active as far as possible.

— **Get through something:**

i. *consume, use a certain amount.* He gets through 40 cigarettes a day.

ii. *pass an exam, test.* Marvellous. I've got through my Final FRCS.

— **Get through to someone:**

i. *make contact, communicate.* We are in despair. We just can't get through to our son at all.

ii. *reach, especially by telephone.* I've tried six times to speak to Dr Varley at St Mary's but I can't get through.

— **Get together:** *assemble, meet.* The Management and the Union should get together to settle this problem.

— **Get up:** *rise from bed.* Do you have to get up in the night to pass water?

— **Get up to something:** *do something surprising or unacceptable.* My parents have no idea what I get up to.

GIVE

— **Give something back to someone:** *restore, return.* The operation should give you back the use of your legs.

— **Give in (to someone/something):** *stop arguing, fighting, trying, etc.* Mrs Spearey was marvellous. She had so much illness but she would not give in.

— **Give out:**
  i. *come to an end* (of food supplies, strength, etc.). I can't go on any longer. My strength has given out.
  ii. *fail, stop working.* At the end of the 6-hour operation, the patient's heart gave out and he died.
— **Give something out:** *distribute.* Those leaflets must be given out to all staff explaining the new safety regulations.
— **Give someone up:**
  i. *renounce hope.* The doctors had given her up months ago but she made a marvellous recovery.
  ii. *stop having a relationship with someone.* Why don't you give him up if he treats you so badly?
— **Give something up:** *stop doing something.* (a) How can I give up smoking? (b) I used to be a teacher but I gave it up last year.

GO

— **Go against something:** *conflict with something.* Private medicine goes against the principles of the NHS set up in 1946.
— **Go ahead with something:** *proceed with something.* I've decided I want to go ahead with the operation.
— **Go along with someone/something:**
  i. *accompany.* Nurse, go along with Mrs Hooper to the X-Ray Department, will you?
  ii. *agree.* I can't go along with your idea of a further operation.
— **Go at someone:** *attack physically or verbally.* I was walking down the street and a young man went at me, knocked me to the ground and took my bag.
— **Go back:** *return.* I want you to go back to your GP with this letter.
— **Go by:** *pass (of time).* As time goes by, you'll get used to wearing the artificial limb.
— **Go by something:** *form an opinion.* I know I look well but that's nothing to go by. I feel terrible.

— **Go down:**
  i. *be swallowed* (of food and drink). My food won't go down (i.e. I have difficulty swallowing food).
  ii. *be reduced in size, level, etc.* How's your ankle? Well, the swelling has gone down but it's still very painful.
  iii. *become lower, fall* (of prices, temperature, weight, etc.) (a) His temperature has gone down. (b) I used to be 9st 7lbs and then I had an ulcer and went down to $8\frac{1}{2}$ stones. (See page xi.)
  iv. *decrease in quality, deteriorate.* Standards of behaviour have gone down in recent years.
— **Go down with something:** *become ill with something.* All the children have gone down with measles.
— **Go for someone:** *attack physically or verbally.* She went for him with a knife.
— **Go for someone/something:** *Fetch.* Go for Sister, quickly.
— **Go in for:**
  i. *enter for an examination.* Hundreds of doctors go in for the FRCS every year.
  ii. *study for a particular profession.* Are you going in for medicine like your father?
— **Go into something:** *investigate.* The Paediatric Intensive Care Unit has been closed while the authorities go into the sudden deaths of ten babies.
— **Go off:**
  i. *deteriorate, get worse.* Her work has gone off since the accident.
  ii. *explode.* She had to have plastic surgery after an oil heater went off in her face.
  iii. *faint, fall asleep, lose consciousness.* (a) If he sees blood, he goes off. (b) It takes me ages to go off. Sometimes I take a sleeping pill.
  iv. *go bad* (of food or drink), *become unfit to eat or drink.* The food poisoning was caused by eating some meat that had gone off.
  v. *stop* (of pain). I've had this abdominal pain for a month. When I take the tablets it goes off, but it comes back.

— **Go off someone/something:** *to lose one's liking or taste for someone/something.* (a) My wife's gone off me. (Usually means does not wish to continue sexual relationship.) (b) I've gone off drink since my operation. (c) I've gone off my food completely.

— **Go on:**

    i. *continue.* (a) This trouble with your bowels has been going on for years, hasn't it? (When followed by a verb, it is in the – ing form.) (b) Go on taking the tablets. (c) Should I go on working while I'm pregnant, Doctor? It is often used negatively: (d) I can't go on any longer like this. Can you give me something to help me, Doctor?

    ii. *happen, take place.* What's going on?

— **Go on something:**

    i. *begin to receive payments from the State because of unemployment.* We've had to go on social security as we've no other money coming in.

    ii. *go on the pill; begin to take the contraceptive pill.* When did you first go on the pill?

— **Go on at someone:** *to complain of someone's behaviour, work, etc.* He never stops going on at me.

— **Go out:**

    i. *be extinguished* (of fire, light, etc.). All the lights have gone out.

    ii. *leave the house.* (a) I'm longing to go out again. (b) You should be able to go out in a couple of days.

— **Go over something:** *check, inspect details, repeat.* Well I've told you what the treatment involves and I'm going to go over it again to make sure you understand.

— **Go round:** *spread from person to person* (of illness). There's a nasty virus going round at the moment.

— **Go round to:** *pay a visit locally.* I went round to see my GP last week and he sent me here.

— **Go through:** *endure, experience, suffer.* (a) When did he go through the phase of passing enormous stools? (b) She's gone through a very bad patch recently (an unhappy or difficult time). (c) I can't tell you what I've gone through since my husband died.

— **Go under:**

　i. *have an anaesthetic*. The patient went under at twelve and came round at four o'clock.

　ii. *die* (slang). Do you think he's going to go under?

— **Go up:** *rise* (of blood pressure, temperature, etc.). Your blood pressure has gone up again.

— **Go with someone:** *accompany*. Have you anyone who can go with you to hospital?

— **Go without something:** *manage without something*. (a) I have to go without food before I have the barium enema. (b) They went without sleep for several days.

KEEP

— **Keep away from someone/something:** *avoid being near to*. Keep away from anyone with German measles if you are pregnant.

— **Keep someone/something back:** *hold back*. (a) My disability will never keep me back. (b) She couldn't keep back her tears.

— **Keep someone down:** *dominate, oppress*. They had a difficult childhood. Their father kept them down.

— **Keep something down:**

　i. *keep something in the stomach* (often used negatively meaning to vomit). She's so thin because she can't keep anything down.

　ii. *not increase something* (e.g. wages, prices, weight, etc.). (a) Keep your weight down. (b) Restricting salt in the diet may help keep blood pressure down.

— **Keep someone from doing something:** *prevent*. All this coughing keeps me from sleeping.

— **Keep off something:** *not drink, eat, smoke, etc*. (a) Keep off fatty foods. (b) You must keep off alcohol while you're taking these tablets.

— **Keep on doing something:** *continue doing something, do* *something repeatedly*. The majority of women in the UK keep on working nowadays. (NB: keep doing something has the same meaning as keep on doing something.) Michael keeps getting stomach cramps.

— **Keep to something:** *adhere to an agreement, a course, a diet, etc*. Keep to the diet for another two months and then we'll see how you are.
— **Keep someone up:** *prevent someone from going to bed*. The baby kept us up all night with his crying.
— **Keep one's spirits, strength up:** *not allow to fall*. (a) She is a very brave woman and always keeps her spirits up. (Remains cheerful.) (b) You must eat to keep your strength up.
— **Keep up with someone/something:** *move, progress at the same rate*. Elderly people find it difficult to keep up with all the changes of modern life.

LET

— **Let someone down:** *disappoint, fail to help*. I can't go into hospital Doctor. I can't let my children down.
— **Let up:**
    i. *become less intense, severe*. If only this pain would let up for a while.
    ii. *relax one's efforts*. After the train crash, the doctors worked night and day to treat the injured. Finally, they were able to let up a little.

LOOK

— **Look after oneself/someone:** *take care of*. (a) She is old and frail and needs to be properly looked after. (b) Who will look after your children when you come into hospital?
— **Look after something:** *be responsible for*. The laboratory technicians look after the equipment and keep it in good order.
— **Look at something:** *examine carefully*. I want to look at your ear to see what's causing the trouble.

— **Look down on someone/something:** *feel superior.* Her husband looks down on her because she hasn't been to university.

— **Look forward to doing something:** *think of something in future with pleasure.* I'm looking forward to having this plaster off.

— **Look in:** *make a short visit to someone's house.* The stoma nurse will look in again next week.

— **Look into something:** *investigate.* We must look into this complaint. It says someone was left lying on a trolley in the corridor for one hour without being attended to.

— **Look on:** *watch something without taking part.* Whilst the surgeon performed the delicate operation, doctors from many countries looked on.

— **Look on someone/something:** *consider.* He's looked on as the most eminent surgeon in this field.

— **Look out:** *be careful, watch out.* Look out! You'll burn yourself on that stove.

— **Look out for someone/something:** *watch carefully for someone/ something.* When examining patients, doctors look out for physical signs prevalent at particular ages.

— **Look over:** *inspect buildings, papers, etc.* Can you look over this report before I submit it to the Working Party?

— **Look through something:** *examine papers quickly.* I'll just look through the notes before seeing the next patient.

— **Look to someone/something:** *take care of.* The child-minder looks to the children while I'm at work.

— **Look up:**
    i. *improve.* How's Mrs Cox? Oh, she's looking up.
    ii. *raise eyes.* Open your eyes now and look up. I'm going to put some drops in your eyes.

— **Look someone up:** *visit someone, especially after a long time apart.* Do look me up when you next come to London.

— **Look something up:** *search for a word, fact in a reference book.* If you don't understand the colloquial English your patient uses, look it up in the Manual.

— **Look up to someone:** *admire, respect.* Most patients like to look up to their doctors.

MAKE

— **Make something of someone/something:** *understand the nature or meaning of someone/something.* (a) We don't know what to make of this change in her behaviour. (b) What do you make of it all?

— **Make off with something:** *to steal something and run away with it.* The youth made off with the drugs he'd found.

— **Make someone out:** *understand someone's behaviour.* We just can't make Mary out at all. She's changed so much since she left home.

— **Make something out:**
    i. *manage to read.* Can you make out what this letter says?
    ii. *manage to understand.* We'll have to get an interpreter. We just can't make out what this patient says.
    iii. *write a cheque, a prescription, etc.* The doctor made out a prescription for my asthma.

— **Make up:** *apply cosmetics.* Whenever I make up, I come out in a rash all over my face.

— **Make something up:**
    i. *invent a story, especially to deceive someone.* Stop making things up. What really happened?
    ii. *prepare a bed.* Keep the patient here. The bed hasn't been made up yet.
    iii. *prepare medicine.* Take this prescription to the pharmacist and he'll make it up for you.
    iv. *supply deficiency.* It's not harmful to be a blood donor. The loss of blood is made up quite quickly in a healthy person.

— **Make up for something:** *compensate.* No amount of money can make up for the loss of her husband.

PUT

— **Put something aside:** *save money, etc., for future use.* Everything costs so much these days. I can't put anything aside for my old age.

— **Put someone away:** *to confine someone to prison or mental hospital* (often used in passive). (a) The old man began to wander in the street at night so his family put him away. (b) He was put away for 20 years for rape.

— **Put something away:** *save money for future use.*

— **Put something back:**
   i. *drink large amount of alcohol* (slang). He must have put back a lot of beer to be in this state.
   ii. *impede.* The accident has put back his hopes of climbing Everest.

— **Put something by:** *save money for future use.* Have you anything put by?

— **Put something down:**
   i. *kill animal because it is old or sick.* I had to have my dog put down last week.
   ii. *place a baby in bed.* I put him down at nine and he starts crying at eleven.
   iii. *write down.* I'd better put down when to take the tablets or I shall forget.

— **Put something down to:** *consider something is caused by.* What do you put this rash down to, Doctor? I put it down to an allergy.

— **Put something forward:** *propose, suggest.* At the meeting it was put forward that more operations should be dealt with in the Day Surgery Unit.

— **Put something in:**
   i. *install.* We aim to put a CT scanner in every hospital by 2000.
   ii. *spend time on work.* Junior doctors often put in over 12 hours' work a day.

— **Put in for something:** *apply for a job.* He's put in for over 20 jobs without any success.

— **Put someone off (something):** *disturb, upset.* (a) He could never be a doctor. He's easily put off by the sight of blood. (b) Food just puts me off at the moment.

— **Put someone off doing something:** *dissuade someone from doing something.* My parents tried to put me off living with Tom but I took no notice.

— **Put something off:** *delay, postpone.* The operation had to be put off because the patient developed a chest infection.

— **Put something on:**
  i. *get dressed.* You can put your clothes on now, Mrs Turner.
  ii. *increase weight.* Good. You've put on six pounds since we last saw you. (See page xi.)

— **Put someone out:**
  i. *anaesthetise.* They put me out and I came round three hours later (slang).
  ii. *annoy, upset.* She was put out because her doctor didn't explain what the procedure involved.

— **Put something out:**
  i. *dislocate.* I think you've put your shoulder out and we must X-ray it to be sure.
  ii. *extinguish fire, light.* Firemen soon put the fire out.

— **Put someone through:** *connect on telephone.* Put me through to A and E, will you please?

— **Put someone up:** *provide a bed and food.* I lost my job and my home. A friend put me up for a few weeks but I'm homeless again.

— **Put something up:**
  i. *increase price.* My landlord has put the rent up by £10 a week so I'll have to go.
  ii. *raise.* The pain's so bad I can't put my arms up to do my hair.

— **Put up with someone/something:** *bear, tolerate.* (a) I'm afraid there's not much they can do about this condition. I'll have to put up with it. (b) How did she put up with that violent husband for so long?

RUN

— **Run across someone/something:** *to meet someone or find something by chance.* I've never run across this before. I think it's a case of botulism.

— **Run away from someone/something:** *suddenly leave, escape.* He's always been a difficult child. He ran away from home at the age of six.

— **Run someone/something down:**
   i. *hit and knock to the ground.* The cyclist was run down by a lorry.
   ii. *speak badly about someone.* He's always running down his wife in public.

— **Run someone in:** *arrest and take to police station.* He was run in for burglary with violence (slang).

— **Run into something:**
   i. *collide or crash into.* A man has just been brought into A and E. He ran his car into a wall in the fog.
   ii. *get into danger, debt, trouble, etc.* We've run into debt and my husband's drinking heavily.

— **Run something off:** *make copies on a machine.* Could you run off twenty copies of this hand-out, please?

— **Run out of something:** *come to an end* (of permits, supplies, time, etc.). (a) Make sure we've enough clean pyjamas this weekend. We mustn't run out. (b) I'm nearly 80 you know. I'm running out of time. (c) My energy is running out.

— **Run over someone:** (of a vehicle) *knock someone down and pass over body.* He's been run over and has broken his ribs.

— **Run over something:** *read quickly, repeat.* Will you just run over the facts again?

— **Run through something:**
   i. *discuss, examine, read quickly.* I've run through the names of patients admitted this week but your son's is not there.
   ii. *spend carelessly, wastefully* They have run through thousands of pounds on advertising.

  iii. *use up*. We run through a lot of disposable gloves in the gynaecological clinic.

— **Run up something:** *accumulate bills*. Why did you run up such large bills?

SEND

— **Send for someone:** *tell someone to come*. He's failing. Send for the ambulance.

— **Send for something:** *order something to be delivered*. Send for two hundred disposable syringes, will you please?

— **Send off something:** *post*. Don't forget to send off those letters today.

SET

— **Set aside something:**
  i. *save money for particular purpose*. She sets aside a bit of money every month to pay her fuel bills.
  ii. *keep time for a particular purpose*. You must set aside half an hour a day to practise the relaxation exercises.

— **Set back someone/something:** *delay progress of someone/something*. (a) Mr Deakin was making a good recovery after his operation but unfortunately a complication has set him back. (b) Work on the new theatre has been set back three months.

— **Set in:** *begin and seem likely to continue* (of infection, rain, winter, etc.). (a) When cold weather sets in, the elderly must take precautions to care for themselves. (b) You can see gangrene has set in to your left leg and as it has not responded to treatment we have no alternative but to remove it.

— **Set on someone:** *attack*. I got this bite when a dog set on me.

— **Set someone up:** *make better, healthier*. A week by the sea will set you up after the hysterectomy.

TAKE

— **Take after someone:** *resemble in appearance or character*.

I'm worried about Jane. She's so different from me. She takes after her father.

— **Take something away:**

i. *cause a feeling, etc. to disappear.* (a) I'll give you some tablets to take the pain away. (b) All this worry has taken my appetite away.

ii. *remove.* They've taken her womb away.

— **Take someone away from someone/something:** *remove.* When sexual abuse was suspected, the children were taken away from their parents on the recommendation of social workers.

— **Take something down:** *record, write something.* Can you take down the history?

— **Take something in:** *absorb, understand by listening or reading.* He was so confused he could not take in what the doctor was saying.

— **Take something off:**

i. *amputate part of body.* His left arm had to be taken off below the elbow.

ii. *have time away from work for special purpose.* I'm taking next week off to be at home when my wife comes out of hospital.

iii. *lose weight by dieting.* You're overweight. I want you to take off a stone. Go and see the dietitian and she'll give you a diet sheet. (See page xi.)

iv. *remove part of clothing.* You needn't take off all your clothes. Just your shirt and trousers.

— **Take on something:** *agree to do work, have responsibility.* Don't take on too much for the next six weeks.

— **Take something out:** *remove or extract.* (a) I must have this tooth taken out. It's giving me a lot of pain. (b) She's going into hospital to have her appendix taken out. (c) We're going to take the stitches out tomorrow.

— **Take something over from someone:** *take control, responsibility from someone else.* Can you take over my bleep for ten minutes while I examine this patient?

— **Take to someone:** *develop a liking for someone.* I never took to my daughter-in-law. She's caused so much trouble in the family.

— **Take to something/doing something:** *begin to do something as a habit.* (a) We need help. Our only son has taken to drugs. (b) He's taken to going for long walks late at night.

— **Take up something:**
  i. *absorb, occupy time.* Medicine takes up all his time and energy.
  ii. *start a job.* We expect you to take up your duties on 1st January.
  iii. *start a profession, hobby, etc.* He's thinking of taking up psychiatry as a career.

TURN

— **Turn against someone:** *become hostile to.* After our divorce, my wife tried to turn the children against me.

— **Turn someone away:** *refuse to give help.* Doctors cannot turn sick people away.

— **Turn someone/something down:**
  i. *reject an idea, person, proposal.* They turned me down as a pilot because of my eyesight.
  ii. *reduce volume of gas, sound, etc.* When they turn down the television I can't hear a thing.

— **Turn in:**
  i. *go to bed* (slang). It's usually two o'clock before I turn in.
  ii. *be pigeon-toed.* He walks with his toes turned in.

— **Turn something in:** *stop doing something* (slang). The job was ruining my health so, although I loved it, I had to turn it in.

— **Turn someone off:** *cause someone to be disgusted by something or not sexually attracted to someone.* His drinking and bad breath turned me off.

— **Turn something off:**
  i. *stop the flow of electricity, gas, etc.* Don't forget to turn off the machine before you leave the building.

ii. *stop radio, TV.* The TV is going all day. He never turns it off.

— **Turn on someone:** *attack.* As I left the building, the guard dog turned on me and bit my leg.

— **Turn someone on:** *give great pleasure, excite sexually.* Psychedelic drugs turn you on very quickly.

— **Turn something on:** *allow gas, electricity, water to flow.* Make sure the computer on which the records are stored is turned on first thing.

— **Turn something out:** *extinguish light or fire.* Please turn out the lights before going home.

— **Turn someone out:** *force someone to leave a place.* I've nowhere to sleep. My partner has turned me out.

— **Turn out:** *prove to be.* I never thought it would turn out to be fatal.

— **Turn over:** *change position of body by rolling.* Turn over onto your left side and draw your knees to your chest.

— **Turn someone/something round:** *face in different direction.* Turn round and let me look at your back.

— **Turn to someone/something:** *go for advice, help.* (a) Hospitals are good places to turn to when you are ill. (b) Sadly, when his wife left him he turned to drink for solace.

— **Turn up:**
   i. *appear, arrive.* Mr Fox hasn't turned up yet for his appointment.
   ii. *be found, by chance, after being lost.* Thank goodness those keys have turned up. We thought they'd been stolen.

— **Turn something up:** *increase volume of radio, TV, etc.* I have to turn up my hearing aid to listen to the news.

TEST PAPER

Complete the following sentences with one word per gap and explain the meaning:

1. I can't finish my work because the computer has broken ......
2. He collapsed in the street and we've been trying to ...... him round for ten minutes.

3. My son's always coming .... colds and flu. I'm worried about him.

4. You've had bronchitis every winter. You really must ...... down your cigarettes.

5. I'd like to see you do ...... your clothes.

6. This constant pain really gets me......

7. How can I ...... up smoking, Doctor?

8. Since the accident he's gone ...... his food and has lost weight.

9. It's difficult for me to keep ...... alcohol.

10. We must ...... into these complaints about long waiting times.

11. Can you get an interpreter? We can't make ...... what this patient is saying.

12. I'm sorry. We'll have to put ...... your operation for a week.

13. Make sure we never ...... out of disposable syringes.

14. Do I need to ...... all my clothes off?

15. I'm getting deaf. I have to turn the TV ...... to hear the news.

16. Get the fire extinguisher. A fire has broken ...... in the office.

17. When I eat shell-fish I ...... out in a rash.

18. My son was terribly cut ...... when he lost his job.

19. We hope you will ...... back the use of your arm soon.

20. I see the swelling on your leg has gone ...... That's good.

Test paper answers

1. break down (fail to work)
2. bring round (resuscitate)
3. come down with (become ill)
4. cut down (reduce amount)
5. do up (button, fasten)
6. get down (depress)
7. give up (stop)
8. go off food (lose appetite)
9. keep off alcohol (not drink)

10. look into (investigate)
11. make out (understand)
12. put off (postpone)
13. run out of (come to end of supply)
14. take off clothes (remove)
15. turn up (increase volume)
16. break out (sudden start of fire etc.)
17. come out in (erupt in rash)
18. cut up (upset)
19. get back (recover)
20. go down (reduce)

Language of drug culture

10

The use of drugs in the UK for recreational purposes continues to grow and to be accepted as normal by many, especially the young. The many different substances being misused, the different ways of taking them and their varying effects present a complex picture. This is reflected in the special language used by many to communicate with other drug users about drugs, drugs equipment and the different stages of effect of the drug.

Of necessity, this language changes frequently and indeed some may only be used in one particular area of the country. The following glossary is a selection of the words and phrases in current use. The abbreviations n (noun) and v (verb) are used.

TYPES OF DRUG

Opioids:
— *DF118:* DFs.
— *Diconal:* Dike.
— *Fortral:* Fortral.
— *Heroin:* Big Harry, Brown, Chi, China white, Dragon, Elephant, Gear, H, Harry, Homebake, Horse, Joy, Junk, Mexican brown, Poison, Powder, Shit, Skag, Smack, Stuff, Tiger, White dynamite.
— *Methadone:* Amps, Juice, Linctus, Phy, Phy pills.
— *Morphine:* Morf.
— *Palfium:* Palf.
— *Pethidine:* Peth.

Stimulants:
— *Amphetamine, methylamphetamine, methedrine:* Nikki, Nose, Nose candy, Speed.

— *Amphetamine sulphate:* Sulph.
— *Blue amphetamine pills:* Blues, Bluies
— *Cocaine:* Bernice, Big C, C, Candy, Carrie, Cecil, Charlie, Cholly, Coke, Corine, Crack (see below), Dust, Freeze, Girl, Gold dust, Happy dust, Ice, Lady, Leaf, Loppy dust, Nose candy, Paradise, Royalty, Sleigh ride, Smack, Snow, Stardust, Toot, White girl, White stuff.
  – *Crack cocaine:* Base, Freebase, Pebbles, Rocks, Scud, Wash.
— *Dexedrine:* Dex, Dexies.
— *Ecstasy:* Adam, Apples, Bunnies, Diamonds, Dick, E, Einsteins, Fantasy, Love dove, MDMA, Rhubarb and custard, Smilers, Strawberries, XTC.
— *Methedrine etc.:* Meth.
— *Preludin:* Prellies.
— *Ritalin, methentermine:* Rit.
— *Stimulants:* Pep pills, Uppers.

Sedatives:
— *Amytal:* Amytal.
— *Barbiturates:* Abbots, Barbs, Blockbusters, Blockers, Blue angel, Blue devils, Christmas trees, Downers, F-40s, Goofballs, Gorilla pills, Green dragons, Idiot pills, Marshmallow, Mexican reds, Neb, Pink ladies, Reds and blues, Sleepers, Softballs, Stumblers, Yellows.
— *Chloral hydrate:* Knockout drops, Mickey Finn.
— *Depressants:* Downers, Sleepers.
— *Doriden:* Cibas.
— *Heminevrin:* Hem, Heminev.
— *Heroin on a barbiturate base:* Red chicken.
— *Librium:* Libs, Greens and blacks.
— *Mandrax:* Mandies.
— *Mogadon:* Mogies.
— *Nembutal:* Nembies.
— *Quaaludes, methaqualone:* Ludes.
— *Seconal:* Seckies.
— *Tuinal:* Tuies.

— *Valium:* Vals.

Psychedelics:

— *LSD:* Acid, Blue star, Californian sunshine, Dots (microdots, LSD), Paper mushrooms, Smiley, Sugar, Tab, Trips, Whizz (tablets impregnated with LSD).
— *Ginseng* (mild Chinese psychedelic, not controlled).
— *Psilocybin:* Magic mushrooms.
— *Serenity, tranquillity, peace:* Peace pills, STP.

Cannabis: Afghan, Bar, Bhang, Black rock, Blond hash, Boo, Brass, Broccoli, Buddha, Bush, Charge, Charlie, Chitari, Dry high, Gangster, Giggleweed, Grass, Hemp, Kif, Malawi grass, Panama red, Shit, Spliff (cannabis cigarette). Stuff (cannabis and heroin), Temple balls, Thai sticks, Yesca, Zani.

Cannabis/Marijuana: Hash, Lebanese gold, Acapulco gold (high-quality cannabis), Sausage, THC, Resin (cannabis), Brick (kilo of compressed marijuana), Dope, Mary Jane, Pot, Weed, Tea, Grass (all marijuana), Ganga (West Indian hashish), Joint, Smoke, Blo, (cannabis cigarettes), Roach (the end part of a joint containing the cardboard support), Mellow (dried banana skins for smoking). Seeds, Pearly gates (morning glory seeds).

Marijuana cigarette: African woodbine, Drag, Joint, Joystick, Reefer, Sausage (Musicians), Smoke, Stick. Blast party: group of marijuana smokers smoking together. Blast a stick: smoke a marijuana cigarette. Blow a stick: as above. Block: black market term for ounce of hashish (resin). Bun: quantity of cannabis resin, Burn (n): a solitary minor smoking of marijuana. Deal: small amount of cannabis. Fingers: cannabis resin. Manicure: clean and prepare marijuana for rolling into cigarettes. Pot-head: marijuana user. Rolling-up: making a marijuana cigarette. Skins: papers to roll joints and make reefers or joints with. Smoke (v): to smoke marijuana cigarette. Stoned: marijuana effect. Teahead: user of marijuana. Turn on (v): to smoke a marijuana cigarette. Weed Heads: marijuana users. Wrap up: brown paper packet containing cannabis.

Solvents: Nose-bag, Spray, Stick-up.

DRUG TAKERS: THEIR EQUIPMENT, HABITS, ETC.

Acid Head: regular user of LSD.

Amp: ampoule, a container of dangerous drugs.

Arrow: injection equipment.

Bad hit: an undesirable effect after taking a drug.

Bagman: drug supplier.

Banger: hypodermic needle.

Barbed up: intoxication with barbiturates.

Binge, going on a: to go on an intensive period of drug taking.

Biz: equipment for injecting.

Bongs: glass smoking pipes.

Brew up: prepare an injection.

Burn (v): to take someone else's narcotic and not return it, to smoke (mainly marijuana).

Business: injecting equipment.

Cap: capsule of narcotics.

Carry (n): a load of drugs.

Chasing the dragon: (a form of free-basing) heating heroin on tinfoil and inhaling fumes.

Clean: recovered from drug dependence.

Connection: dealer in narcotics.

Cook up: prepare for an injection.

Crank up: to inject a narcotic.

Cut: adulterate narcotics.

Dealer: person from whom drugs are obtained.

Dirty fix: unhygienic injection.

Doctor Scrip: a doctor who easily prescribes drugs.

Doobs: pills.

Dope: any narcotics.

Drop (v): to swallow a pill.

Drug free: recovered from drug dependence.

Fix (n): an injection.

Fix (v): to inject a drug.

Flushing: drawing blood back into syringe and injecting back into vein.

Free-basing: method of purifying street drugs (e.g. chasing the dragon, smoking crack).

Gear: addict's drug.

Gimmicks: equipment for injecting.

Glue-sniffing: practice of inhaling vapour from glue and other volatile substances such as butane gas, petrol, etc.

Guide: someone familiar with drugs and relatively sober while others try it for the first time.

Gun: equipment for injecting.

Habit: addiction to drugs with physical dependence; dosage commonly taken.

Hard stuff: cocaine and opiates.

Hippy: drug user, especially psychedelic.

Hit: experience injection.

Hooked: addicted to drugs.

Hustling: buying drugs.

Ice cream habit: irregular drug habit.

Jab: inject drugs.

Jack up: take an injection of a narcotic.

John: lavatory, place for injecting.

Jolt: inject drugs into vein.

Junkie: heroin taker.

Kit: drug addict's equipment.

Lady: glassware for smoking cocaine.

Load (n): stock of illegal drugs.

Loaded: full of drugs.

M.: morphine.

Machinery: equipment for injecting.

Mainlining: injecting intravenously.

Middle man: dealer in narcotics.

Mumbling: conning or tricking the doctor.

Nail: needle.

Needle: addict's syringe, etc.

Okay scene: enjoyable drug party.

On look out: searching for drugs.

Outfit: drug addict's equipment.

Peddler: seller of drugs.

Pill head: person on pills, usually amphetamine type.

Pipes, to do: smoke crack in pipes.

Pop: inject.

Popping: subcutaneous injection of a drug.

Pusher: person who sells drugs illegally and tries to induce people to start taking them.

Quill: folded matchbox cover for sniffing narcotics through the nose.

Registered: obtain regular prescription for drugs.

Rip off (v): to smoke.

Runner: drug supplier.

Scene: place where people meet to take drugs, group of users of drugs, particular group of people.

Score (v): to obtain drugs.

Scrip, Script: a prescription for drugs.

Set of works: addict's syringe, etc.

Shoot up: take an injection.

Shooting gallery: place where addicts meet to shoot up.

Shot: an injection.

Sink (v): to swallow a pill.

Skin-popping: subcutaneous or intramuscular injection.

Sniff (v), Snort (v): to sniff narcotics through nose, usually heroin or cocaine.

Snowballing/Speedballing: injecting or sniffing a mixture of heroin and cocaine.

Spike: hypodermic needle.

Stash: hiding place for narcotics.

Stuff: any narcotics.

Stuffer: smuggler who conceals drugs in anus or vagina to avoid detection.

Supplier: drug source.

Suss out: police search for drugs.

Swallower: person who swallows drugs (e.g. in a condom) to avoid detection.

Tabs: tablet form of drugs, usually LSD.

Tie up: tourniquet used to prepare vein for injection.

Tools: addict's apparatus.

Tracking: injecting intravenously along a vein.

Turn on (v): to give a non-addict his first shot.

Turned on: under the influence of drugs.

User: taker of drugs, mainly narcotic.

Works: addict's apparatus.

LANGUAGE USED TO EXPRESS EFFECTS OF DRUG TAKING

Bad trip: bad experience from LSD.

Bang, Buzz, Flash, Rush: sensation experienced after injecting a narcotic intravenously.

Be heavy, serious (v): to be heavily addicted.

Blasted: under influence of drugs.

Blocked: being under the influence of a drug (particularly drinamyl).

Blow your mind (v): to enter into a frenzied state of mind.

Bombed: high on drugs.

Brought down (v): to be elated and then suddenly unexpectedly depressed.

Bummer: unpleasant experience, especially with LSD.

Buzz: effect induced by taking drugs.

Charged up/coasting: under the influence of drugs.

Come down (v): to lose drug-induced exhilaration as it wears off.

Come up (v): experience of drug working.

Crash: sleep, pass out from drugs.

Experience: LSD or mescaline experience.

Flake out (v): to lose consciousness.

Flash: effect of cocaine; to lesser extent of methedrine.

Freak out: bad experience from LSD.

Gouch (v): be high on heroins.

Groove/Grooving: having a good time on drugs.

High: feeling good; state of euphoria after taking drugs.

Horrors: acute unpleasant drug effects: (i) cocaine or amphetamine psychosis; (ii) acute withdrawal.

Kick: effect of drug, particularly a stimulant.

Nod (to nod, on the nod): drowsy state following injection of narcotics.

Off your face: high on drugs.

Pinned: description of constricted pupils after consuming heroin.

Psychedelic experience: effect of LSD or other hallucinogen.

Raver: person under influence of excessive amount of amphetamine.

Red eye: refers to conjunctival infection. May occur after use of marijuana.

Rush: the euphoric effect of a drug on the user.

Spaced out: out of touch with reality.

Stoned (v): to be under influence of drugs.

Taste (a taste of): taking a small amount of a drug and having little reaction.

Track marks: signs of injection in veins.

Trip: effect of LSD or other hallucinogen.

Turned on: under the influence of drugs.

Wired to the moon: high on drugs.

Wrecked: high on drugs.

LANGUAGE OF WITHDRAWAL

Catch up: to withdraw from drugs.

Cleaned out, Dried out: drug free, to have taken a 'cure'.

Clear up: to withdraw from drugs.

Clucking: withdrawal from opiates/opioids.

Cold turkey: Abrupt withdrawal of narcotics. Derived from appearance of skin — usually called 'goose flesh'.

Detox: give up drugs; withdrawal under medical supervision.

Drying out: slow withdrawal from narcotics.

Fold up: withdraw from drugs.

Hung up: unable to get drugs, depressed, let down, disappointed.

Kicking the habit: stopping drugs.

Make the turn: withdraw from drugs.

Munchies: to eat excessively when being withdrawn from narcotics.

Shakes, Sick: narcotic drug withdrawal symptoms.

Strung out: feeling ill from lack of narcotics or other hard drugs.

Turned off: withdrawn from drugs.

Washed up: withdrawn from drugs.

GENERAL SLANG USED BY ADDICTS

(Slang word in bold type)

Bad scene: unpleasant surroundings, bad situation, bad vibrations.

Big house, in the: in prison.

Big John: the police.

Bird, 'to do bird': to serve a prison sentence.

Boxed: in prison.

Bread: money.

Brief: warrant to arrest or search.

Buff: money.

Bull: detective.

Bum: tramp.

Bust (v) (busted): to arrest (to be arrested).

Canned: to be arrested.

Champ: drug user who will not reveal his source.

CID: detective.

Clean: off narcotics, not carrying drugs at that time.

Cop out: confess.

Croker: doctor.

Croker joint: hospital.

Derry: derelict house.

Dibble: police.

Dirty money: money from crime/drugs.

Fall: to be arrested.
Fink: informant.
Freak: a long-haired drug user.
Fuzz: police.
Gas: terrific, marvellous.
Grass: informer.
Groovy: up-to-date, beautiful, good.
Hang up: personal problem.
Hassle: inconvenience, nuisance.
Heavy: important, serious.
Heeled: possessing drugs.
Hot: wanted by police.
Hotload: overdose which may be fatal.
Jugged: to be arrested.
Junkie: drug addict.
Kip (v) (to have a kip): sleep (not always rough).
Laundering money: A process to hide the criminal source of money and make it appear legitimate.
Law: policeman.
Man: police authority.
Meths: methylated spirits.
Mule: carrier of drugs for another, usually over international borders.
Nicked: arrested.
Old Bill: policeman.
On Ice: in prison.
On the bricks: released from prison.
Pad: room, or apartment.
Pass: a transfer of drugs or money.
Pig: policeman.
Plain clothes: detective.
Plant: hiding place or cache of drugs.
Porridge: prison term.
Pulled: to be arrested.
Rat: to go back on a bargain or inform on someone.
Rave: acid house party or pay party.

Reader: prescription.

Red Biddy: methylated or surgical spirits in wine (N. Ireland).

Rip off: sell weak or non-narcotic substances as hard drugs.

Road: on the road, vagabond life.

Rumble: police nearby.

Scratch: money.

Shrink: psychiatrist (head shrinker).

Skippering: travelling about with one's belongings, bedding down with others.

Sleep rough: sleep anywhere.

Square: conventional, old-fashioned, not 'with-it'.

Squat: illegal occupation of premises.

Stash: hide drugs.

Stool: informer.

Straight: ordinary tobacco cigarettes; a non-drug user.

Time (doing time): to serve a prison sentence.

Toss: search a person or premises.

Travel agent: street drug dealer.

Turkey: poor quality drugs or non-drug substance used to deceive.

Turn over (v): to rob.

Uptight: angry, tense, worried.

Wrap: street quantity of drugs sold in small paper bags etc.

Medical abbreviations

11

The rapid development of medicine and the related sciences in recent years has brought a vast increase in medical vocabulary. At the same time, the increased speed of life has driven people to use abbreviations more and more and this tendency is well illustrated in the medical and scientific field.

Abbreviations are disliked and discouraged by many doctors because they are variable and misleading. The choice between capital and small letters and the use of the full stop (e.g. A.C. rather than AC) is often a personal one. The same initials may have different meanings in different medical fields.

Nevertheless, abbreviations *are* used every day in medical reports, on record cards and case histories and in speech, and a knowledge of them is, therefore, absolutely essential.

A SELECTION OF ABBREVIATIONS COMMONLY USED BY THE MEDICAL PROFESSION IN THE UK

A

A – acute; anterior; artery; attendance

A₃, A₇ – to attend surgery in three, seven days

aa – (Greek: of each) used to show the same quantity of each ingredient in a prescription

AAS – anthrax antiserum

ABG – arterial blood gas

AC – air conduction; alternating current; anodal closure

a.c. – ante cibum (Latin) before meals

ACE – angiotensin converting enzyme

ACTH – adrenocorticotrophic hormone

ADH – additional duty hours; antidiuretic hormone

ADL – activities of daily life

A & E – Accident and Emergency Department

Aet – aetas (Latin) age

AF – atrial fibrillation

AFB – acid fast bacilli

AFP – alpha fetoprotein

A/G ratio – albumin/globulin ratio

AI – aortic incompetence; aortic insufficiency; artificial insemination

AID – artificial insemination by donor

AIDS – acquired immune deficiency syndrome

AK – above knee

Alb – albumin

ALL – acute lymphoblastic leukaemia

ALP – alkaline phosphatase

ALT – alanine transaminase

Amb – ambulance

AML – acute myeloid leukaemia

AMOH – Association of Medical Officers of Health

amp – ampere; amputation

AN – antenatal

ANF – antinuclear factor

ANS – autonomic nervous system

AP – anteroposterior; artificial pneumothorax

APH – antepartum haemorrhage

APN – artificial pneumothorax

ARC – AIDS-related complex

ARF – acute renal failure

ARM – artificial rupture of membranes

AS – alimentary system; anxiety state; aortic stenosis

ASD – atrial septal defect

ASO – antistreptolysin O

AST – aspartate transaminase

ATN – acute tubular necrosis

AVC – atrioventricular canal

AVM – atrioventricular malformation

A & W – alive and well

AXR – abdominal X-ray

AZT – azidothymidine (Zidovudine)

Å – angstrom unit

B

B – brother

Ba E – barium enema

Ba M – barium meal

BB – bed bath; blanket bath

BBA – born before arrival

BBD – baby born dead

BCG – bacille Calmette Guérin

b.d. – twice a day

BF – breast fed

BI – bone injury

BID – brought in dead

b.i.d. – bis in die (Latin) Twice a day

BIH – bilateral inguinal hernias

BK – below knee

BM – bowel movement

BMA – British Medical Association

BMI – body mass index

BMR – basal metabolic rate

BNA – Basle Nomina Anatomica

BNF – British National Formulary

BNO – bowels not opened

BO – body odour; bowels opened

BOR – bowels opened regularly

BP – blood pressure; British Pharmacopoeia

BPC – British Pharmaceutical Codex

BPD – biparietal diameter

BPH – benign prostatic hyperplasia

Br – bronchitis; brown

BRCS – British Red Cross Society

BS – breath sounds; blood sugar

BSE – bovine spongiform encephalopathy

B'sp – bronchospasm

B Wt – birth weight

C

C – carbon; cathode; centigrade (temperature scale); certificate; cervical; consultation

C 1 – 8 – cervical spine segments

CAPD – continuous ambulatory peritoneal dialysis

CBD – common bile duct

Cf – first certificate

C₁, C₄, C₁₃ – intermediate certificate for 1, 4, 13 weeks

CF – final certificate

Cp – private certificate

c. – circa (Latin) about

c. – with

Ca – carcinoma

CAL – chronic airways limitation

CAO – chronic airways obstruction

CAPD – continuous ambulatory peritoneal dialysis

CBT – cognitive behaviour therapy

CC – chest clinic; creatinine clearance

cc – cubic centimetre

CCF – congestive cardiac failure

CD – Controlled Drugs

CDH – congenital dislocation of hips

CF – cardiac failure; cystic fibrosis

CFA – cryptogenic fibrosing alveolitis
CFS – chronic fatigue syndrome
CFT – complement fixation test
CGD – chronic granulomatous disease
Cgh – cough
Ch – child; children; chronic
CHD – congenital heart disease
Cho/Vac – cholera vaccine
CI – colour index
CIN – cervical intraepithelial neoplasia
Circ – circulation; circumcision
CJD – Creutzfeldt Jakob disease
CLA – community living assessment
cm – centimetre
CMV – cytomegalovirus
CNS – central nervous system
CO – Casualty Officer
C/O – complains of
COAD – chronic obstructive airways disease
C of H – circumference of head
Comp – complemented
Conj – conjunctivitis
COOP – care of older people
COP – change of plaster

COPD – chronic obstructive pulmonary disease
CP – colour perception
C'p – chickenpox
CPAP – continuous positive airways pressure
CPD – cephalopelvic disproportion
CPK – creatinine phosphokinase
CPR – cardiopulmonary resuscitation
CRF – chronic renal failure
CRP – C-reactive protein
CSA – child sexual abuse
CSF – cerebrospinal fluid
CSM – Committee on the Safety of Medicine
CSSD – Central Sterile Supply Depot
CSU – catheter specimen of urine
CT – computerised tomography
CV – cardiovascular; cervical vertebra; colour vision; conversational voice; curriculum vitae
CVA – cerebrovascular accident
CVP – central venous pressure
CVS – cardiovascular system; chorionic villus sampling
Cx – cervix
CXR – chest X-ray
Cyl – cylinder
Cz – coryza

D

d – density; dioptre; dorsal; dose

D/ – daily total in divided doses

D 1 – 12 – dorsal spine segments

DA – dental anaesthetic

DAO – Duly Authorised Officer

D & C – dilatation and curettage

DCR – dacro-cysto-rhinostomy

D & D – drunk & disorderly

DED – date expected delivery

Derm – dermatitis

Dh – dermatitis herpetiformis

DH – drug history; Department of Health

DIC – died in Casualty; disseminated intravascular coagulation

Dip – diphtheria

Dip/Vac/FT – diphtheria prophylactic formol toxoid

DLE – disseminated lupus erythematosus

DMO – Divisional Medical Officer

DMR – Duty Medical Registrar

DN – district nurse

DNA – deoxyribonucleic acid; did not attend

DNKA – did not keep appointment

DNS – deflected nasal septum; did not suit

DOA – dead on arrival

DOB – date of birth

DOM – Dept. of Medicine

DOS – Dept. of Surgery

DP/Vac – diphtheria pertussis prophylactic vaccine

DPP – diphtheria pertussis prophylactic

DS – disseminated sclerosis; double strength

D Sph – dioptre spherical

DSR – Duty Surgical Registrar

DT – delirium tremens; diphtheria and tetanus; distance test

DT/Vac – diphtheria tetanus vaccine

DTN – diphtheria toxin normal

DTP – diphtheria, tetanus and pertussis

DU – duodenal ulcer

Dup – duplicate

DV – domiciliary visit

DVT – deep venous thrombosis

D & V – diarrhoea and vomiting

DXR – deep X-ray radiation

DXT – deep X-ray therapy

Dysm – dysmenorrhoea

Δ – diagnosis

† – died

E

E – evening
EAA – extrinsic allergic alveolitis
EBS – emergency bed service
EBV – Epstein–Barr virus
ECF – extracellular fluid
ECG – electrocardiogram
ECT – electroconvulsive therapy
EDC – expected date of confinement
EDD – expected date of delivery
EDM – early diastolic murmur
EEG – electroencephalogram
EENT – eyes, ears, nose and throat
EMU – early morning specimen of urine
ETT – examination in theatre
ENT – ears, nose and throat
EOM – external ocular movement
ERCP – endoscopic retrograde cholangiopancreatography
ERPC – evacuation of retained products of conception
ES – enema saponis
ESM – ejection systolic murmur
ESN – educationally subnormal
ESR – erythrocyte sedimentation rate
ESRD – endstage renal disease
ETT – exercise tolerance test
EUA – examination under anaesthesia
Ez – eczema

F

F – Fahrenheit (temperature scale); father; female
FA – fatty acid; fibrosing alveolitis
FB – foreign body
FBC – full blood count
FBS – fasting blood sugar
FDP – fibrinogen degradation products
FFP – fresh frozen plasma
FH – family history; fetal heart
FHH – fetal heart heard
FHNH – fetal heart not heard
FHSA – Family Health Services Authority
Fib – fibrositis; fibula
f.m. – fiat mistura (Latin) make a mixture
FMF – fetal movement felt
FMP – first menstrual period
FP – food poisoning
FPC – family planning clinic; family practitioner committee
FT – formol toxoid; full term
FTA – fluorescent treponemal antibody

FTBD – fit to be detained; full term born dead

FTND – full term normal delivery

FVC – forced vital capacity

FW – forced whisper

G

γ **GT** – gamma glutaryl transferase

g – gram(s); gramme(s)

GA – general anaesthetic; general attention

G and A – gas and air

GB – gallbladder

GBM – glomerular basement membrane

GC – general condition; gonococcus

GCFT – gonococcal complement fixation test

GFR – glomerular filtration rate

GH – growth hormone

GI – gastrointestinal

GIFT – gamete intrafallopian transfer

GIT – gastrointestinal tract

GMC – General Medical Council

GORD – gastro-oesophagitis reflux disease

GP – general practitioner

GPC – general physical condition

GPI – general paralysis of the insane

G6PD – glucose-6-phosphate dehydrogenase

GTT – glucose tolerance test

GU – gastric ulcer; genitourinary

Gyn – gynaecology

H

H – hospital, hydrogen

HA – Health Authority

Hb – haemoglobin

HBD – hydroxy-butarate dehydrogenase

HC – head circumference; hydrocortisone

HDL – high-density lipoprotein

HF – Hageman factor

HI – head injury

HIV – human immunodeficiency virus

HLA – human leucocytes antigen

H of F – height of fundus

HM – head movements

HNPU – has not passed urine

HP – House Physician

HPC – history of presenting complaint

HR – heart rate

HRO – Hospital Resettlement Officer

hrs – hours

HRT – hormone replacement therapy

HS – heart sounds; House Surgeon

Ht – heart; height

H/T – hypertension

I

IBS – irritable bowel syndrome

ICF – intracellular fluid

ID – infectious disease

IM – intramuscular

Impr – improved

INR – international normalised ratio

IOFB – intraocular foreign body

IP – inpatient; insurance patient; interphalangeal

IQ – intelligence quotient

IRL – infrared light

IRU – industrial rehabilitation unit

ISQ – in status quo

ITU – intensive therapy unit

IU – international unit

IUD – intrauterine device

IU(C)D – intrauterine contraceptive device

IV – intravenous

IVC – inferior vena cava

IVF – in vitro fertilisation

IVP – intravenous pyelogram

IVU – intravenous urogram

IVUD – intravenous urodynamogram

IZS – insulin zinc suspension

J

JVP – jugular venous pressure

K

KUB – kidney, ureter and bladder

L

l – litre

Ⓛ – left

L 1–5 – lumbar spine segments

Lab – laboratory

LA – left atrium; local anaesthetic; local authority

LAD – left anterior descending (of coronary artery); left axis deviation

LAH – left anterior hemiblock

lb – pound (of weight)

LBBB – left bundle branch block

LBP – low back pain

LCA – left coronary artery

LDA – left dorsoanterior position of the fetus

LDH – lactic dehydrogenase

LDL – low-density lipoprotein

LDP – left dorsoposterior position of the fetus

LE – left eye

LE cells – lupus erythematosus cells

LFA – left frontoanterior position of fetus

LFP – left frontoposterior position of the fetus

LHA – Local Health Authority

LIF – left iliac fossa

LIH – left inguinal hernia

LLL – left lower lobe

LLZ – left lower zone

LMA – left mentoanterior position of fetus

LMC – local medical committee

LMN – lower motor neurone

LMP – last menstrual period; left mentoposterior position of fetus

LMZ – left middle zone

LOA – left occipitoanterior position of fetus

LOP – left occipitoposterior position of fetus

LP – lumbar puncture

LPH – left posterior hemiblock

LSCS – lower segment Caesarean section

LSE – left sternal edge

LUA – left upper arm

LUZ – left upper zone

LV – left ventricle; lumbar vertebra

LVA – left visual acuity

LVF – left ventricular failure

LVH – left ventricular hypertrophy

M

M – male; malignant; morning; mother

mane – in the morning (of drugs); tomorrow

MAIC – mycobacterium avium intracellulare

M and CW – maternity and child welfare

M/F; M/W/S – male/female; married/widow(er)/single

Mc – millicurie(s)

MCA – Medicines Control Agency

MCH – mean corpuscular haemoglobin

MCHC – mean corpuscular haemoglobin concentration

MCL – mid-clavicular line

MCV – mean corpuscular volume

MDM – mid-diastolic murmur

ME – myalgic encephalomyelitis

mEq – milliequivalent(s)

MHO – Medical Health Officer

MI – mitral incompetence or insufficiency; myocardial infarction

Misc – miscarriage; miscellaneous

MM – multiple myeloma

MMR – mass miniature radiography
MO – Medical Officer
MOH – Medical Officer of Health
MOM – milk of magnesia
MOP – medical outpatient
MR – manual removal; mitral regurgitation
MRC – Medical Research Council
MRI – magnetic resonance imaging
MRSA – methicillin resistant staphylococcus aureus
MRU – Mass radiography unit
MS – mitral stenosis; multiple sclerosis; musculoskeletal
MSU – mid-stream urine
MSW – Medical Social Worker
mμ – millimicron(s)
MWO – Mental Welfare Officer
M.XR – mass X-ray
μ – micron
μg – microgram(s)

N

N̄ or **Ⓝ** – normal
NA – National Assistance; not applicable
NAD – no abnormality detected
NAH – not at home
NAI – non-accidental injury

NBI – no bone injury
ND – normal delivery; not diagnosed; not done
NE – not enlarged
NFA – no fixed abode; no further action
NFV – no further visit
NG – new growth; no good
NGU – non-gonococcal urethritis
NI – National Insurance
NIC – National Insurance Certificate; National Insurance Contributions
NIL – not in labour
nocte – in the evening (of drugs)
NK – not known
NM – neuromuscular
NMR – nuclear magnetic resonance
NND – neonatal death
NOTB – National Ophthalmic Treatment Board
NP – nomen proprium
NPU – not passed urine
NS – nervous system; not seen
NSAID – non-steroidal anti-inflammatory drug
NSPCC – National Society for the Prevention of Cruelty to Children
NSU – non-specific urethritis
N & T – nose and throat
N & V – nausea and vomiting
NYD – not yet diagnosed

NYK – not yet known

O

OA – occipitoanterior; osteoarthritis
OAP – old age pensioner
Occ – occasionally
OD – overdose
ODQ – on direct questioning to systems review
O/E, OE – on examination; otitis externa
OM – omne mane (every morning); osteomyelitis; otitis media
ON – omne nocte (every evening)
Op – operation
OP – occipitoposterior
OPA – outpatient appointment
OPD – outpatients department
OT – occupational therapy; old tuberculin
OTC – over the counter – drugs bought without a prescription from a doctor

P

P – pulse
PA – pernicious anaemia; posteroanterior; pressure area; pulmonary artery
Paed – paediatric
PAN – polyarteritis nodosa
Para – 0 + 0 (2 + 1) Formula meaning: P (number of pregnancies); a (number of abortions); ra (number of living children); no live pregnancy + no non-viable pregnancy; (two live children + one non-viable)
PAT – paroxysmal atrial tachycardia
PBI – protein bound iodine
PBZ – phenylbutazone
PCN – percutaneous nephrostomy
PCNL – percutaneous nephrostomy lithotomy
PCP – pneumocystis pneumonia
PCR – polymerase chain reaction
PD – peritoneal dialysis
PDA – patent ductus arteriosus
PE – pulmonary embolus
PEEP – positive end expiratory pressure
PEFR – peak expiratory flow rate
Pen – penicillin
PET – positron emission tomography; pre-eclamptic toxaemia
PFR – peak flow rate
PGL – persistent generalised lymphadenopathy
PH – public health
pH – symbol for expression

of hydrogen ion concentration

Phy – pharyngitis; physician

PHLS – Public Health Laboratory Service

PI – principal investigator; pulmonary insufficiency

PID – pelvic inflammatory disease; prolapsed intervertebral disc

PL – perception of light

PM – postmortem

PMB – postmenopausal bleeding

PMH – past medical history

PMP – previous menstrual period

PMT – premenstrual tension

PN – postnatal

PND – paroxysmal nocturnal dyspnoea

p.o. – per os (Latin) by mouth

PO, P Op, Post-op – postoperative; postoperation

POP – Plaster of Paris

PP – private patient

PPD – progressive perceptive deafness

PPH – postpartum haemorrhage

PR – per rectum

p.r.n. – pro re nata (Latin) as required

Prem – premature

PS – per speculum; pulmonary stenosis

PSM – pansystolic murmur

Pt – patient

PT – physical training; pulmonary tuberculosis

PTA – prior to admission

PTB – pulmonary tuberculosis

PTSD – post-traumatic stress disorder

PTT – partial thromboplastin time

PU – passed urine; peptic ulcer

PUO – pyrexia of unknown or uncertain origin

PUVA – photochemical ultraviolet light – A waves

PV – per vaginam

PVT – paroxysmal ventricular tachycardia

PZI – protamine zinc insulin

Q

QALY – quality adjusted life year

q.i.d. – quater in die (Latin) four times a day

q.d.s. – four times a day

R

R – red; respiration

R – recipe (Latin) take (used in prescriptions)

Ⓡ – right

RA – rheumatoid arthritis; right atrium

RAD – right axis deviation

RBC – red blood cell count; red blood corpuscles

RBS – random blood sugar

RDA – recommended daily allowance

RE – right eye

Rh – Rhesus factor; rheumatism

RIF – right iliac fossa

RIH – right inguinal hernia

RLL – right lower lobe

RLZ – right lower zone

RML – right middle lobe

RMO – Regional or Resident Medical Officer

RMZ – right middle zone

RNA – ribonucleic acid

ROA – right occipital anterior

ROO – Resident Obstetric Officer

ROP – right occipital posterior

ROS – removal of sutures

Rpt – repeat; report

RR – respiratory rate

RS – respiratory system

RSO – Resident Surgical Officer

RTA – road traffic accident

RTI – respiratory tract infection

RUA – right upper arm

RUL – right upper lobe

RUZ – right upper zone

RV – residual volume

RVA – right visual acuity

RVH – right ventricular hypertrophy

S

S – schedule e.g., S 4 – schedule iv Poisons; single dose; sister

S 1–5 – sacral spinal segments

SAD – seasonal affective disorder

SAE – stamped addressed envelope

SAH – subarachnoidal haemorrhage

SARE – serum angiotensin converting enzyme

Sat – satisfactory

SB – stillborn

SBE – subacute bacterial endocarditis

SC – subcutaneous

SEN – State Enrolled Nurse

SG – specific gravity

SGOT – serum glutamic oxaloacetic transaminase

SGPT – serum glutamic pyruvic transaminase

SH – social history

SI – sacroiliac; schedule 1; soluble insulin; statutory instrument

SIDS – sudden infant death syndrome

Sig – signa (Latin) label (in prescriptions)

SLE – systemic lupus erythematosus

SM – systolic murmur

SMO – Senior Medical Officer

SMR – submucous resection

SN – student nurse

Sn – Snellen test type

SNO – Senior Nursing Officer

SOA – swelling of ankles

SOB – short of breath

SOBOE – short of breath on exertion

SOL – space-occupying lesion

SOP – surgical outpatients

SOS – supplementary ophthalmic service

Spec Gr – specific gravity

Spt – spirit; sputum

S (R) – single dose – usually repeated 2 or 3 times in the day

St – stone (of weight)

Stat – immediately (refers to administration of drugs)

STs – sanitary towels

STD – sexually transmitted disease

Sub – subsequent dose

Sulpha – sulphonamide

SVC – superior vena cava

SVD – simple vertex delivery

SVT – supraventricular tachycardia

SWD – short-wave diathermy

Sy – syphilis

Syph – syphilis

T

T – temperature; term; treatment

T 1–12 – thoracic spine segments

TA – triple antigen

T & A – tonsils and adenoids

TAB – typhoid – paratyphoid A and B vaccine

TABC – typhoid – paratyphoid A, B and C vaccine

TAB/Cho – typhoid – paratyphoid A + B vaccine + cholera vaccine

TABT – typhoid – paratyphoid A and B vaccine with tetanus toxoid

TB – tuberculosis

TBM – tuberculous meningitis

TCA3(7) – to come again in three (seven) days

TCI – to come in

TENS – transcutaneous electrical nerve stimulation

Tet – tetanus, tetracycline

Tet/Ser – tetanus antitoxin

Tet/Vac – tetanus toxoid

Tet/VacFT – tetanus toxoid

Th V – thoracic vertebra

3TC – antiretroviral drug – lamivudine

TI – tricuspid incompetence

TIA – transient ischaemic attack

t.i.d. – ter in die (Latin) three times a day

t.d.s. – three times a day

TN – temperature normal

TOP – termination of pregnancy

TPI – treponemal immobilisation test

TPR – temperature, pulse, respiration

TPV – triple polio vaccine

TR – temporary resident

TS – tricuspid stenosis

TSH – thyroid-stimulating hormone

TT – tetanus toxoid; tuberculin tested

TTA – to take away ⎱
TTH – to take home ⎬ refers to drugs
TTO – to take out ⎰

TV – trichomonas vaginalis

U

U – unit

U and E – urea and electrolytes

UG – urogenital

UGS – urogenital system

UGT – urogenital tract

UMN – upper motor neurone

URTI – upper respiratory tract infection

U/S – ultrasound

UTI – urinary tract infection

UVA – ultraviolet A

UVB – ultraviolet B

UVL – ultraviolet light

V

V – visit

V 10 – visit in 10 days

VA – visual acuity

Vac – vaccination

Vag – vaginitis

VD – venereal disease

VDRL – Venereal Disease Research Laboratory

VDRT – venereal disease reference test

VE – vaginal examination; varicose eczema

VF – ventricular fibrillation

VI – virgo intacta

VRE – vancomycin resistant enterococci

VSD – ventricular septal defect

VT – ventricular tachycardia

VU – varicose ulcer

VV – varicose vein(s)

Vx – vertex

W

W – weekly dose

WBC – white blood cell count; white blood corpuscles

WC – water closet = lavatory; whooping cough

WR – Wassermann reaction
Wt – weight
WVS – Women's Voluntary
   Service

X

X – multiple
XR – X-ray

Xs – excess

Y

yr – year

Z

ZA – Zondek–Aschheim
ZN – Ziehl–Neelsen